THE
TIME MACHINE
DIET

To Michelle,
with best
wishes

June 8, 2021

ISBN: 978-0-9737796-7-7 (paperback)
ISBN: 978-0-9737796-6-0 (eBook)

Published by Reality Trader Services

Editing: Katrina Asselbora, Mark Ierardo
Cover Design: Iryna Spica
Typeset in *Abril Text* at SpicaBookDesign

Printed in Canada by Printorium Bookworks / Island Blue, Victoria B.C.

To my Dad.
I wish I could have written this book
thirty years ago.

Alarm Bell

Diabetes – the best thing that ever happened to me.

Bet you don't hear that every day.

Meanwhile, this is exactly how I feel 3 years after being diagnosed with Type 2 Diabetes. Had this alarm not sounded loud as thunder, would I change radically the way I eat? In all likelihood, I would still be a heavy sloth: severely obese, out of breath when walking up any incline, taking medication for high blood pressure and heartburn, and slowly deteriorating – all the while coming up with excuses for being badly out of shape. "It's genetics, it's age, my metabolism slows down, I don't eat all that much..." They provide great comfort – and remaining in the comfort zone guarantees that nothing will ever change.

Hearing my alarm bell loud and clear, I dropped the excuses that might have made me feel better but wouldn't help me change a thing. I did my homework and took action. Today I am seventy five pounds lighter, eight inches thinner at the waist, in a great physical shape and off medications. Health wise, I traveled back in time 25 years, to the 30-years old version of myself. Thank you diabetes for waking me up!

Whether you have had your own alarm bell or not (and I hope you haven't and won't), you can benefit from my experience. Prevention is the best medicine. Trying to fix something after it breaks is much, much harder. Let this book help you avert your wake-up call. Better to read a book and take action than get diagnosed with diabetes or cardiovascular problem, don't you think?

The methods I used and described in this book can help you dramatically improve your well-being and physical shape while adding absolutely delicious foods to your menu. They are common sense and they feel natural. Give them a shot!

Table of Contents

SECOND PRONG: PLUS BACTERIA

THIRD PRONG: MINUS POUNDS

Follow the author's journey
through weight loss to a medication-free life using
modified eating patterns and delicious foods

THE
TIME MACHINE
DIET

Travel back to your naturally
healthy energetic self

Vadym Graifer

STARTING POINT

Shocked Into Reality

I don't know why this question surprised me so much. It really shouldn't have. After all, my lineage forewarned me that I was all but destined to have it. Being overweight should have added to the grave acknowledgement that I was bound to find myself there one day. Yet I was shocked and incredulous. What was this weary looking doctor reading my bloodwork sheet talking about?

– For how long have you had diabetes?

I don't have diabetes! I had my blood tested last time, when?... Was it two years ago? Three? No, two. It was fine! I am here because of this pesky kidney stone, that's all.

– Doc, what diabetes? I don't know anything about that. Haven't had any signs... could it just be the pain caused by the stone that distorted the reading?

The good doctor sighed and nodded – a nod that I grossly misinterpreted at the time. I took it as "yes, it's a possibility." Knowing what I know now I would have decoded it as "here is another poor soul in denial, walking around undiagnosed, and blissfully unaware of the grave consequences, destined to take ever-increasing doses of the medications, never having the strength to change his whole lifestyle, all but certain to deteriorate slowly, start insulin injections in a few years and see his quality of life constantly declining." Tough verdict, isn't it? Yet this is exactly the image you project when you say "What diabetes? I don't have diabetes!"

– Follow up with your family doctor, get that blood sugar checked and go from there, okay?

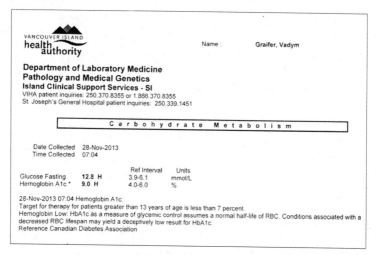

BLOOD GLUCOSE READING AT THE DIAGNOSIS

So I did. Sure enough, the doc didn't sigh for nothing. My A1C was at 9%. If you are a diabetic, you know the meaning of that number. If not (and hopefully this book will help prevent you from becoming one), the simple explanation is: Anything above 6.5% is diabetes, and above 7% – poorly controlled diabetes. Oh, and a fasting blood sugar reading at 12.8 mmol/l (that's 230 mg/dl for

US readers) didn't help either – that's at least twice the norm. The verdict was in.

Let me step back for a minute and tell you how I got there. My Dad was diagnosed with diabetes at the age of 46. His condition deteriorated steadily, and he passed away at 68, having lost his sight and being home-bound for the last few years. His Dad had diabetes, and had his foot amputated in his 60s. That gives you an idea of my family's predisposition. I had fought my tendency for weight gain since I was in my mid-thirties. "Fought" is merely a figure of speech here, as proven by my clueless eating habits – drinking pop, a cup of tea with 3-4 teaspoons of sugar, pastry here and largish piece of cake there, bread, pasta, rice, pizza. At 5 ft. 10 in. tall, I got myself to 260 pounds by the age of 40.

In case you prefer a metric system, one pound is ~0.45 kg, and one kg is ~2.2 pounds. So, those 260 pounds translate into 118 kg. See Resources for the most common unit conversions in this book.

Diagnosed with hypertension and feeling badly out of shape, I finally got the message and started the long quest to lose weight. Cutting down on sugar and processed food, decreasing my carbs consumption and increasing my physical activity, I managed to lose about 30 pounds over the next couple of years. Moving from Winnipeg to Victoria, BC with its much milder climate opened the possibility of year-round outside activity and helped me lose another 5-7 pounds. Then I decided to get even healthier and quit smoking (yeah, with all that family history and all that weight I was also stupid enough to continue smoking from my teen years). That was a great decision in many respects, but my weight exploded back up to 250 pounds before I regained some control and managed to stop the relentless march upward. A low carb/high protein diet took me down to about 230, and for the next year or two I was slowly drifting up to 240 and down to 230, depending on wind direction, star alignment, and who knows what else (you can see the thread of denial familiar to many overweight folks, right?) So, that's where the diabetes diagnosis found me: 52-years old, about 240 pounds, taking Chlorthalidone (a water pill) for my blood pressure, apple-shaped with a lot of abdominal fat and on the last hole of my 46-inch belt.

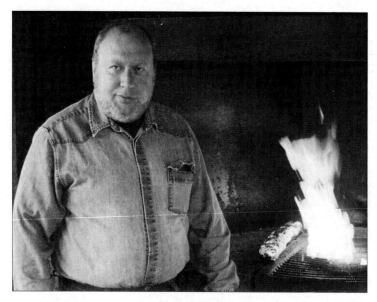

AT 260 POUNDS

Is this situation rare or unique in any way? By no means. I won't overburden you with statistics – I know the media bombards us with horrifying numbers about obesity and diabetes every day of the week. If you haven't heard those, you must be living on some other planet, in which case you are unlikely to read these pages either. So I will safely assume that you are well aware of just how many of us walk around with one or both of these maladies (and in all likelihood a few more). Moreover, if you have decided to read this book, chances are you or someone close to you is in a similar predicament. Chances are, you struggled with your situation for a while and found out just how difficult it is to take it under control. Chances are, you sensed that with all of the medical science advances, it's ultimately up to you to use them effectively and change your life. Finally, chances are you sought help in structuring your approach to your health, reconciling all the conflicting bits and pieces of information we get from every direction, and you could use the real life experience of someone who successfully navigated those stormy waters. If all of this sounds true to you, read on to see how the approach described in this book helped me and what you can expect from it.

Journey, Briefly

Let me describe the journey I took so you can gauge the steps involved and the approximate timelines. My ambition was not merely to manage my weight and disease; it was to try and reverse my Type 2 diabetes.

> *The definition I used for "reverse" has been given by Ann Albright, PhD, RD, the director of Division of Diabetes Translation at the Centers for Disease Control and Prevention: "The term 'reversal' is used when people can go off medication but still must engage in a lifestyle program in order to stay off." The concept of "lifestyle change" sat just fine with me since it was obvious that my previous way of life was headed toward a dead end – pun intended.*
>
> *You may find the concept somewhat debatable, as indeed many in the medical profession do. Such a definition, for instance, doesn't outline the time needed to confirm the reversal; some insist on six months, some prefer one year, or other arbitrarily picked period. There is scarce data available indicating the likelihood of relapse over various periods of time. One view is that if you can stay in the healthy range with no medication for the duration from one A1C test to another twice (6 months) and the lifestyle that gets you*

there is sustainable, you have achieved the reversal, or remission. Its permanency is in your hands, however, as you are likely to remain in "at risk" group. If down the road for whatever reason you veer off course and fall "off the wagon" again, triggering the return of diabetes – that's your own negligence which by no means diminishes the effectiveness of the method that brought you to remission. Nor can such improvement of your condition be a bad thing, so don't let those doubts stop you. If the word "reversal" makes you uncomfortable, let's call it "getting your test results in a healthy range." To sum it up, the view I subscribe to is: If your numbers indicate non-diabetic range and you can maintain this state without medications and unsustainable restrictions to your diet, the goal has been achieved, whether you call it reversal, remission or (stretching it a bit) cure. You will find a few interesting links discussing this topic in the Resources.

The whole undertaking took me about two years, from the first steps described in the book to reaching my ideal weight, dropping blood pressure medication and getting my diabetes in remission. That happened three years after getting diagnosed as I spent the first year or so feeling my way around, researching numerous approaches and methods and familiarizing myself with the basics.

Seeing myself at 240 pounds, with a 46 inches waist, an A1C at 7.5 and continuously increasing dose of Metformin, I finally started formulating the first stage of what eventually became the three-pronged approach presented in this book. Here is the illustration of that point:

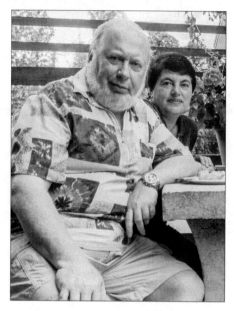

AT 240 POUNDS

Over the next year and a half I implemented what eventually became the first two prongs of my approach. Replacement of the remaining sugary and starchy foods by their healthier equivalents in my daily menu and the introduction of fermented foods obviously helped. My weight started coming down slowly but steadily. Signs that my health was improving were manifesting as well. My weight dropped to 216, for a decent 24 pounds loss. My waist slimmed down to 44 inches, shaving off two inches of abdominal fat. In the fall of 2015 I even finally managed to get my A1C under 7 in two consecutive readings.

However promising these developments were, they remained incremental, not enough to change the situation dramatically. I still was on the medications and still seriously overweight (actually, let's not fool ourselves: with a BMI at 31, it's obese). Nor were these improvements sustainable yet, as over the winter my A1C reading went to 7.3 again, indicating that my control over blood sugar levels remained shaky.

At this point my research took me to the idea of Intermittent Fasting. Over the past few years, this method has showed great potential for facilitating steady and sustainable weight loss. Most of all, records of diabetes reversal were abundant in both medical studies and personal stories floating all over the Internet. In March of 2016, I started this program alongside my wife. Over the next three months I lost 27 pounds, weighed in at 189 pounds and attained an A1C reading of 6.3 – very impressive drop over such a short time.

For the first time since my diagnosis my dose of medication went down. My waist size dropped to 40 inches (a four inch improvement over three months.)

The rate of weight loss was steady and sustainable. The strategy was easy to follow with relatively few sacrifices. My BMI dropped to 27.1, as I moved from the "obese" category to just "overweight." My blood pressure improved dramatically as well, dropping to a healthy 117 over 72. There was also significant improvement in lipids, confirming a substantial progress in overall health.

The following months saw further steady weight loss. By the end of November I hit my target weight of 165 pounds, achieving a 75 pound weight loss since the initial diagnosis and 50 pounds loss over the course of Intermittent Fasting. My waist size dropped to 36 inches (8 inches decrease) and BMI to 23.7 – normal weight territory.

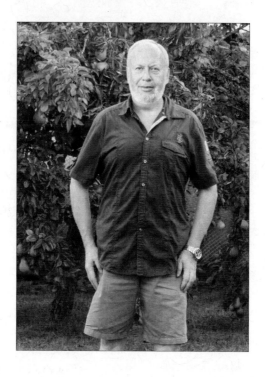

Most important of all, my A1C reading dropped to 6, allowing me to minimalize my Metformin with perspective to drop it altogether. Over these same six months my wife lost 37 pounds, her BMI dropping from 30.1 to 24.2. We both stopped taking our medications for blood pressure control as it stayed in a normal range with no help now. At this point we moved to maintenance mode, which was intended to preserve all the achievements while having, within reason, practically no forbidden foods. We both felt great, getting rid of all of the little pains and aches, feeling fit and energetic. It was as if the time machine took us back to earlier versions of ourselves, back to the time when we were lean, healthy and energetic and needed no drugs. That's when we dubbed our regimen The Time Machine Diet.

As you see, it took about two years for me, but this doesn't mean that it should take this long for you. I was plotting my path step by step, researching, making mistakes and taking detours. Having the benefit of my experience and using this book as a guide, you can walk this path at a much faster pace.

Hopefully, this brief storyline makes you feel encouraged and curious enough to dig into the details and start planning your own journey to a similar destination.

The Three Prongs of
the Time Machine Diet

First of all, let's define "diet" in the framework of this book. The most often used definition of this word in health-related topics, from the Oxford dictionary is: "a special course of food to which one restricts oneself, either to lose weight or for medical reasons." As in "I am going on a diet." In our case, though, another definition fits better: "the kinds of food that a person habitually eats." While we do modify our eating patterns and some foods, the Time Machine approach doesn't entail the usual restrictions you would expect from a diet beyond the exclusion of the outright unhealthy stuff. Nor does it include a meal plan where you get instructed what to eat each day at each mealtime.

Now let me describe the major principles applied in the approach we discuss in this book.

There is one common thread in all the diets that almost invariably fail in the long run. With the exception of the tiniest sliver of the population (we call them supermodels), they can't be sustained in the long run. At best, we can keep them over the course of a few months. Then we go off course, try to climb back on board, fall off again – only to find a new diet and repeat the whole frustrating cycle. Losing some weight, ballooning back up and adding some more is the all-too familiar path for many of us. There are a few reasons for such consistent failures. Formulating these reasons helped me shape up the method that avoids the typical traps of many diets. The major attribute of the right approach, in my view, should be this: it must be natural, matching the way our bodies and minds were designed to work.

This motive will manifest itself in most aspects of the Time Machine Diet, by approximating the suggested way of life to the one that is natural to us by design. It concerns the foods we eat and the foods we avoid, the eating pattern and ways to exercise. There is a certain reassuring elegance in the idea that to travel back in time to the healthier version of ourselves we need to travel back in time and restore the ways we ate centuries or millennia ago. While not exactly a popular lately Paleo type of a diet, it certainly has some common traits with those.

First of all, any diet forbidding whole classes of foods can't be sustained in the long run. There are no bad macronutrients per se: protein, fat, carbohydrates – they all have their role, and banning any of them is not something a healthy way of life should include. No pizza forever? No single piece of bread, ever again? No mashed potatoes or french fries for the rest of your life? No full fat ice cream? Hah! Thus, my approach may loosely regulate certain ratios and suggest certain desirable additions or replacements, but as far as excluding foods, anything goes is the ideal approach. (*Notable exception here is arti-ficially created foods and drinks that carry no nutritional value, have nothing to do with the way our body is intended to work, and often possess addictive qualities that bring nothing but harm.*)

Next, any diet making you a bean counter of cal-ories and grams of various nutrients is likely to cause resentment at some point. Thus, those ratios mentioned above should be loose and intuitive. If any weighing and counting is involved, it should occur during the first steps when we retrain our bodies and restore a natural sense of what is good for us and what is excessive. Veering off those ratios on occasion should not cause guilty feelings; in fact just the opposite should happen – you should feel good about being able to deviate occasionally, and still maintain your healthy way of life.

That takes us to the next extremely important trait of a good program. Few things make your life as glum as constantly fretting about the types of food you eat. Any diet that makes us feel gloomy is destined to fail. Thus, ours must be joyful. If we get rid of some unhealthy, yet tasty ingredient, we need to find a good replacement for it. If we want to introduce some new dish to our diet, it should be tasty and the process of making it should be fun. At no point in our journey did I or my wife feel mis-erable about what we did. It was and remains an exciting endeavour, making us feel curious about the process and encouraged by the results. In fact, we exchanged puzzled glances every time someone told us that we must have had a strong will and great self-control. Nothing of that ever came into play as we enjoyed every minute of it. You don't need a strong will or self-control to do what you enjoy doing. Even the lack of results during some stages was perceived as a motivation to look for more effective strategies. I really hope the book turns out to be contagious in communicating this sense of excitement and generating the same in you.

> *A few more words about motivation. I have to admit, I have difficulty understanding the very concept of needing strong motivation to improve your health. Doesn't a chance to prevent or reverse cardiovascular disease or diabetes, look and feel your best, constitute the strongest possible motivator of all? If such a prospect doesn't inspire you, nothing I could say will.*

The process itself must be exciting, interesting and pleasant. You should be able to enjoy the journey, not merely tolerate it for the sake of the result. Think of it this way: when a good surgeon performs a complicated procedure, does he focus on the surgery itself or on the monetary reward for it? And if he is mostly concentrated on the money he is going to receive for this operation, do you want to be his patient? Focus on doing it right – and the result will follow naturally when you master the process. That's why in good Japanese schools new archers learning the craft start their practice with no target, shooting at an empty wall; they need to master the right form and mindset before focusing on hitting the target. With the right form, precision comes naturally. Thus, make sure you do each and every step with unhurried curiosity, soaking up the process and relishing all the progress – and then enjoying the result that comes seemingly by itself.

Another important aspect is the time expenditure required to lead the advocated way of life. Most of us don't have the luxury of allocating a few hours each day to stay healthy. If I suggest a regimen including hours of cooking and exercising in a gym, it's not likely to sound acceptable even in theory. Thus, nothing in this book demands any significant additional time above what you in all likelihood do anyway. No recipe is too complicated or time-consuming. No physical exercise demands you go to the gym with specific equipment (but neither forbids it if that's what you enjoy). If some of the food preparations feel a bit too involved (those are likely to be some of the fermented foods), it happens at the very beginning only, as you master new things. In a few days as they become routine, they take minutes. Healthy ways of living should be easy and natural, not something labored and duct-taped onto our daily activities. Simplicity and low time commitment is a virtue. We should be able to focus on living our life to its fullest, while the basic maintenance of our ability to function properly should be just an ordinary aspect, not a matter of major attention. Heightened attention, research and effort are justified while we fix the damage caused by years of neglect; a maintenance regime should be as close to an automatic routine as possible.

Along with time required goes the rigidity of the prescribed way of life. Can you complete things on your own schedule or must you keep some rigid timetable? We lead complex lives with a lot of commitments, obligations and constraints. Being able to move your diet's requirements around to fit into all those restrictions makes all the difference. Flexibility is a necessary trait of a good diet. Such a diet also must accommodate the occasional situations where you deviate from all the restrictions so you don't become "that guy" at Thanksgiving dinner – you know, the type that refuses the mashed potatoes with gravy, cranberry sauce and stuffing, and turns away the pumpkin pie, serving as a living reproach to the rest of the guests.

At this point you are probably wondering: Wait a minute, with no limitations on what to eat, no meal plans, schedules, strict portion control and specific recipes, it doesn't sound like a diet at all. Bingo! A good diet that is sustainable, joyful and healthy is no diet at all. It's a way of life that is natural and free-flowing. And that's exactly what we strive to achieve. If any limitations exist in the process, they should be short-lived and easily tolerated. Such limitations are necessary because years of neglect require some repair, but you don't want to live in a state of permanent renovation. You fix things and lead normal life – just don't confuse normal life for causing the damage again. The good news is, if the repair is done correctly you won't even want to return to previous habits, since your body is going to be much more attuned to what's good for it. That's another reason for absence of meal plans of any kind in the book. The lifestyle I advocate entails enjoying various foods and spontaneity, not a structured schedule of meals prescribed and planned in advance.

With all the promise of ease, little time required and few restrictions, let's state though: if you are looking for the results with no effort and time whatsoever, you are holding the wrong book. Any such promise would be misleading and fraudulent. The results possible when you dedicate yourself are not the miracle; they are the outcome of your own actions.

Now we can formulate our objective in this whole undertaking. Here it goes:

THE TIME MACHINE DIET MANIFESTO

Once upon a time, long ago, there was a lean, fit, healthy you who didn't even realize that your body required much attention. Nothing ached or annoyed you, everything worked, there were no forbidden foods, and restoration after any excess took almost no time. That all-but-distant-memory-you is still somewhere inside, hidden within the layers of today's you, with all the little aches and annoyances accumulated over the years and accepted as necessary companions of aging. We want to rediscover that former you and let him out of the prison of fat. We want to shed all those pounds, pains and aggravations amassed over years. We want no life-long restrictive diets, no special time-consuming attention to staying healthy, no forbidden foods – just common sense, easy, enjoyable natural living where everything within reason is allowed in sensible moderation, including occasional deviations from "sensible."

Now, let me give you a description of the three prongs of the Time Machine Diet – a breakdown of the topics in the book, to make your navigation easy and help you see how it all is tied together. We will look into how they work together and the role each of them plays.

The first prong described in the **Minus Sugar** part of the book is devoted to food. It starts with a brief overview of the ways sugar sneaks into our diet and goes on to show what we need to cut out and, more importantly, what to replace it with to eat healthier yet still enjoy the taste. Bread, rice, pasta, potatoes – all these things have tasty and healthy alternatives, variations or, sometimes, better ways to prepare them. We will also speak of resistant starches, their role in a healthy nutrition regime and the ways to introduce them in your diet.

The second prong, **Plus Bacteria**, is a topic I consider to be of the utmost importance. It introduces fermented foods, which cultivate healthy gut bacteria that benefit our well-being enormously. Needless to say, each and every one of the foods discussed will be accompanied by detailed recipes and variations with practical advice to prepare them easily and quickly.

The third prong, titled **Minus Pounds**, describes the method of steady and sustainable weight loss that was applied by me, my wife and countless folks all over the world. It goes over the timeline of our Intermittent Fasting journey, depicting in detail everything that happened to our bodies and minds, and summarizing our experiences in a way that will help you chart your own course. Again, practical tips and tricks is our main focus.

These three components come together as a system where each of them works to support and enhance the effects of the other prongs. The first prong's role is two-fold. Getting rid of the added sugar and cutting down on sugary/starchy foods in our diet decreases inflammation and helps us shed first pounds. Its key effect, however, is in the role sugars play in our hunger-satiety cycles. Sugar promotes over-eating and helps increase our caloric intake far above actual need. Taking control of the sugar content in our food, we prepare our body for Intermittent Fasting – our major weapon against excessive weight. Also, the replacement of harmful foods by healthier alternatives awakens our taste for better nutrition and starts our quest to reshape our sustenance.

The second prong promotes overall health in a way few other methods can. It restores something we have lost in our rush to acquire sterile, processed, convenience food. It's our beneficial gut bacteria, the enormous role of which we started realizing only recently. Normalizing digestion is but one function of healthy gut flora. It's difficult to overestimate the effect it has on our lives and well-being. Helping with various processes, it became an organic part of our method and facilitated positive changes in the body.

The third prong serves as a final blow to the pounds and pounds of fat. Amazingly effective in trimming down all the heavy cargo we carry on our bodies, it digs out that lean fit body hiding under the layers of fat. It returns our body function to the way it was designed to work, going through the alternating cycles of fed and fasted states. Under such a natural regimen, fuel taken in during feeding is being burned during fasting. In the absence of a fasted state, we continue taking in more fuel than we need and our body puts the excess away in the form of fat.

Can you use any of the three prongs alone and still benefit from it? Absolutely. Each one of them is hugely helpful and beneficial to your health. Each of them will advance you in your quest for better well-being. My hope, though, is that you will apply all three – if not in their entirety, then at least some elements of them. Together they make it much easier and more effective. Each of them amplifies the effect of others. They also make the result more sustainable. Finally, each of them is just fun.

Yes, you heard it right – pure unadulterated fun. Experimenting with new and delicious foods, discovering your own variations and tastes is an exciting journey even for those who never were into cooking from scratch. There is something infinitely rewarding in unchaining yourself from industrially processed foods. And yes, believe it or not – fasting is fun. It's not a torture when it's done right; it makes you feel good and opens new ways of enjoying even simple daily activities.

Fasting alone will make you slimmer. It's going to be more difficult to do, though, if you still experience blood sugar spikes and crashes, typical for sugar-addicted individuals. Your hunger pangs and food cravings will be stronger, and it will take longer to get them under control. Excessive sugar intake is not the sole reason for weight gain; over-eating is a major contributor to our layers of fat. Sugar, however, enables and promotes over-eating and multiplies its harmful effects. Cutting sugary and starchy foods will make you healthier and cut some pounds. It will decrease the inflammation and promote better cardiovascular health. It's going to improve glycemic response and hormonal balance. By all means, it's worth doing, whether you adopt the rest of the tactics or stop at that. As a stand-alone weight loss strategy, though, it's not likely to work fast enough and ultimately take you to your ideal weight. Thus, combining the two (sugar cutting and Intermittent Fasting) makes a lot of sense and amplifies the effectiveness of both.

Cultivating your gut bacteria with fermented foods will make you healthier and promote numerous positive changes. The benefits it will bring to your body are endless. Whether you add all of the foods described or just some of them, it's an unquestionably significant addition to your regime, not to mention being tasty as well. Yet again, while it supports and promotes weight loss, it alone won't make it happen rapidly enough or take you far.

So, there you go – you may need or want some of the parts of the approach we discuss here. If that's the case, feel free to pick and choose. If, however, you want the concentrated impact of three very powerful strategies interwoven in a way that magnifies their effectiveness and speeds up the desirable changes in your body, apply the whole thing. You may want to do it at your own pace, matching your circumstances. You may pick some of the suggested foods and omit others, or add different ones based on the principles we discuss. You may select a different modification of fasting, and this book does show a few. All this is to say that the whole approach is very flexible and can be adjusted to your purposes, preferences and tastes while still remaining very effective.

About This Book

First of all, let's firmly establish the following: this is NOT intended as medical advice. I am not a trained MD qualified to analyze your particular situation or conduct a scientific study. I am not trying to dispense a recipe to cure diabetes or cardiovascular disease. What I can and try to do is to share my experience of reading numerous studies, sifting through various angles of dealing with the problem, filtering out the nonsensical, useless or outdated advice (and make no mistake, such filtering is very difficult to do in such a specialized field!), and eventually shaping up a practical way to improve my well-being in a major way and defeat the malaise. Needless to say, everything I describe in the book is based on my own experience.

I am not simply describing the definite path to this final result – that would be based on an assumption that your starting point and conditions are the same as mine, that your body reacts in the same way as mine and your improvement can be achieved in exactly the same steps as mine. Such an assumption would be dead wrong. Thus, I describe the various steps and their variations in hope that some of them will suit your situation even if others won't.

I will share my findings along the way, illustrating their results by documenting the changes in my condition. Where I did a lot of research, I will share the sources and summarize what I eventually compiled from them. This way you will be able to apply my approach and use it in its entirety if it works for you – or go to the source and find the variation that suits you better.

One of the crucially important features of this book: I will share various practical tips and tricks that I worked out by trial and error. You see, it's often not enough to get the right concept and even the right technique. There are those little but all-important things that determine the ultimate success – how to tweak the recipe or change the sequence of your steps, how to trick your body into the right response, how to accomplish something in an easier way or sustain some effort with less difficulty. This is especially true for the multi-step, multi-component pro-grams, like Intermittent Fasting. These kinds of tricks can really make all the difference in terms of the result you are trying to achieve.

Again, let me emphasize the following point: Do you need all of the methods and recipes discussed in the book? Not necessarily. You may find out that one of them solves your problem and gets you right to the finish line (and if that's the case, I bet it's going to be Intermittent Fasting, probably the most potent weapon in the arsenal listed here). Still, I am confident that your overall health will benefit from some other parts of the book, such as the introduction to fermented foods and the recipes for healthy alternatives. Those steps lay the foundation for overall well-being and prepare your body for a healthy way of life. Also, sugar addiction (yes, it's a real thing) makes Intermittent Fasting more difficult, so if you suspect this might be your case, you may want to devote a few weeks to flushing the sugar out of your system.

There is one very important thing to understand about the methodology suggested in the book. This is not a one-time fix for weight-related problems, in the hopes of returning to harmful eating habits. Unless you permanently change the way you eat, you will lose weight, then upon returning to your previous lifestyle gain it back and repeat the whole cycle. Instead of returning to the damaging ways that created the problem in the first place, you are better off adopting the new regime – one that keeps you trim and healthy. Committing to a lifelong pattern of eating requires it to be non-restrictive, full of tasty foods and easy on your time. That's exactly what we strive to achieve with the foods introduced in the first two parts. Thus, I hope that you will utilize the book in its entirety, if not using all of the recipes, then at least some of them.

It's also possible that your variation of the disease is not fully reversible, but one of the methods or a combination of them allows you to control it much better and greatly improves your quality of life, possibly helping to decrease your need for medicine or even drop it altogether. That is a great achievement as well – you can lead a high quality life with well-controlled diabetes, with a much richer diet than many sources would have you believe.

Finally, you may have already begun to make some of the changes suggested in this book – for instance, you may have already banished sugary beverages such as soda from your daily routine. If so, you can still skim through the section to glean some of the substitute drinks recommended; they might be unfamiliar to you but their health benefits will contribute to your quest. Also, it can be useful to have a general idea about the applied approach in case you can identify someone in your life that might benefit from it.

You may also find that some of the steps, ideas or concepts in the book sound familiar. Sure enough, if you have done your research on these topics before, you may see familiar approaches. Still, for those who are at the beginning of the journey, we need to start with the basics. We are going to form a solid foundation for later steps, so use your familiarity with the topic to review what you know.

You may want to read the whole book before starting to implement the ideas it discusses. The point here is this: the book's timeline is dictated by my story, but this is not necessarily a sequence you must apply. You need to write your own story. I was navigating these waters blind but, having the benefit of my experience, you can mix and match the bits and pieces of the approach that work for you, and save a lot of time in the process. A description of some of the steps may have its logical place in later parts of the book, while they can be implemented by you much earlier. The best example of this is a section devoted to physical activity. While logically it belongs to the weight loss section rather than to the parts devoted to food, you don't have to wait to implement it until you get to the weight loss regimen. It can and should become a part of your routine from day one.

The steps outlined in the book, wherever possible, are ordered by increased degree of involvement. It means that the initial steps won't require much thinking or time spent. When you start getting more interested in the whole process, when the results provide encouragement and excite you and when you get genuinely interested in nourishing your body in the best possible way, it's going to be easier to get more involved. More than that, you are likely to want to do that and enjoy every step of the way, being proud of every new skill and accomplishment, of becoming more independent and self-reliant as well as of the results. That said, nothing described and suggested in the book demands full time involvement – not even part-time. It all remains at the level of a mild hobby. Many spend this much and more time pounding the treadmill in gyms or eating in fast food restaurants, neither of which you will have or want to do. To give you an idea of the time allotment required: the longest time dedicated to food preparation in the entire book takes me about 40 minutes and needs to be done once a month to feed two people generously.

Finally, I'd like to discuss the range of readers who might benefit from this book. My particular call to action and a major ailment to fight off was diabetes, so I use it as an example and the storyline. By no means are people living with diabetes the only intended audience though. It can serve a purpose for a much wider circle of readers. Two factors make me think and say that.

The first is, sizeable and sustained weight loss is your major weapon against many conditions. This is what we want to achieve, what I have done and want to show you. Obviously, weight loss is beneficial to a much wider and more universal audience than those living with diabetes. It's a long-standing dream for many people who might have pre-diabetes, undiagnosed diabetes or no diabetes at all. If this book can help them succeed in their goal to lose weight, it means fewer people diagnosed with diabetes, fewer people with hypertension, fewer people with heart problems and countless other complications in the future. If we can prevent some of those, all the better.

The second factor is, this book takes a rather holistic approach to weight loss and the restoration of health. By "holistic" I mean well-rounded: Combining sensible physical activity, good eating habits and choosing/preparing good quality foods. Thus, you will feel, look and function better adopting this approach in its entirety or in parts that appeal to you, hopefully even adding some of your own (it's not like I have exhausted the field).

Thus, my hope is that this book first serves as a better health guide, and a weight loss book second, with one of side benefits being reversal or relief of, among other things, diabetes. I am confident that folks with no excessive weight can also greatly benefit from the ideas suggested in the parts devoted to food. My alarm bell happened to be a diabetes diagnosis; hopefully you haven't had and won't have such a health warning, by applying measures described here pre-emptively.

Let's firmly establish one crucially important point for the folks with diabetes or hypertension: Even though our ideal goal is to get rid of the medications you have to take to control your condition, you do not immediately replace your medicine by the measures we are going to discuss in this book. You implement these measures, assess the results and cut down your doses with your doctor's blessing, if and when your blood sugar or blood pressure reading allows. Then you monitor your state with these decreased doses to make sure that effect stays. And, needless to say but let's say it just the same, you consult with your healthcare practitioner along the way. I have seen enough people willing to experiment with their precious health on their own to stress this warning over and over again: No matter what you think you've learned by reading stories and advice on the Internet, do not dismiss your MD. It's all too easy to confuse superficial and often unsubstantiated "knowledge" for medical training. If this sounds contradictory to applying the methods discussed in this book, that's because it is a somewhat controversial topic. It's just about finding the right balance between professional consultation and applying the bleeding edge innovative methods. Let me expand on that.

When you start researching diabetes (and this remains true for many other ailments) by whatever means possible, it's not going to take very long for you to realize that this is not a single-cause, single-track disease. By that I mean that it's not necessarily caused by the same trigger for all of us, it's not always coming to the same "broken body part" so to speak, and it's not developing in the same way for all of us. While there is a large degree of uniformity in symptoms, there are also a large variety of factors contributing to it. There are various links in our endocrine system that may get broken. There are different ways in which our body deals with this condition and in which the condition develops. While medical science has made impressive strides in studying diabetes, the stark reality is this: There is no way our healthcare can deal with each of us individually to the degree required to find out what's wrong in our particular case. Neither can it monitor how your particular body reacts to different influences, and make fine changes based on those influences until the optimal path is found and implemented. While it might be possible with a simpler disorder, it's certainly difficult with diabetes. Thus, it falls to us to learn everything possible about our individual bodies and work out the right combination of actions – while maintaining the basis of the "standard" measures suggested by your MD. Indeed, in all likelihood you will be encouraged by your healthcare practitioner to educate yourself about your disorder, possibly become a member of a support group in your area (many of those provide a lot of great information) and thoroughly monitor the state of your health, writing down the changes and reaction on them. So, let's be smart about this and take advantage of all the resources available to us: Medical advice, latest studies, age-tested practices, experience of the folks who successfully sailed across the sea of data, and most of all – let's use common sense in both filtering out the falsehoods and in careful application of the relevant information.

Let's also understand that we can't expect our doctor to be aware of all the latest findings in the area of fermented foods, gut bacteria and Intermittent Fasting. It's simply impossible for them to stay abreast of such a broad field, especially if it's not their immediate area of expertise. As recently as 15 years ago the medical community was very skeptical about Intermittent Fasting; today, science is firmly on its side, with strong support from the data collected over the years. Front line medical workers don't usually catch up with the latest research quickly; it takes time for the newest findings to disseminate through the long chain. Thus, we must be cognizant of a necessity to find the fine balance between self-education and heeding professional advice.

That said, one thing may quickly clue you in to the fact that your family doctor is not up to speed with modern diabetes research and you should, perhaps, take his or her advice with a grain of salt. Here it is: if you hear "Your diabetes is a chronic and progressive disease and there is nothing you can do about it," you know you are on your own. Don't take it as a verdict; take it as a signal that you are going to have to do it without much help from this particular doctor.

I would like to stress specifically that everything diabetes-related in this book regards type 2, non-insulin dependent diabetes. If you are type 1 or insulin-dependent type 2, you will benefit from the first two parts of the book, but practicing the third part must be coordinated with your healthcare practitioner and done under his/her supervision.

The same can be said about weight loss in general. One doesn't have to go too far to discover endless suggestions about ways to shed the excess pounds. In fact, if you do have some of those to lose, you have likely tried a few of those suggestions. So have I. The approach that eventually worked for me is based on sound research and a constantly growing body of real-life experiences. Following this path, you are going to use a perfect combination of modern science, age-tested techniques and self-guided steps in adjusting it all to your particular circumstances.

Once again, you don't have to follow the exact order of the steps described in the book. Mix and match them as you please. There is nothing to prevent you from applying the Intermittent Fasting method for a steady and rapid weight loss before introducing some of the fermented foods in your diet. The sequence in this book is just my story as I was feeling my way in the dark. Having the benefit of it, you don't have to repeat it exactly. If you take advantage of my experience and apply my findings to streamline your way to success, that's going to be the highest praise for this book.

Along with the practical help is one more crucial aspect of the whole drive to get trim and healthy. See, all the knowledge in the world won't do us much good unless we are perfectly willing to implement it. Forming the right mind set, finding the way to stay motivated, shaping up our whole mental model of the world and our behavior in it is necessary for the ultimate success of this undertaking. Wherever possible, I share my views on these topics, attitudes I have worked out for myself and the angles that helped me stay the course and remain driven and curious.

You are going to see some skeptical remarks about the role the food industry plays in the current state of affairs. Despite those, I would like to say that the book is not intended as an anti-industry manifesto in any way, shape or form. I want to keep it strictly practical; thus let me simply state the fact that our interests as an individual in search of the best nutritional advice are not always aligned with the interests of a corporation in search of maximizing shareholders' value.

I wanted to incorporate references to studies and sources so they would be actually useful instead of just the inserting numbered references that many find annoying. On one hand, a significant number of readers won't care much about all of the scientific findings with their methodologies, numbers and intricacies; they feel that such insertions interrupt the book flow and make reading difficult. These kinds of references also tend to be more useful during the first read; as you return to the book, as I hope you will, in search of a particular step or recipe, they make the text cumbersome and more difficult to navigate.

On the other hand, many feel that they need to make sure that the science is there and want to read the studies for themselves. Thus, I went for this compromise: I leave the text mostly free from links and footnotes, but the Resources section at the end of the book lists the studies, books and websites used, broken by parts and accompanied by a brief description allowing you to gauge whether the link is of interest to you. This way you can use the book according to your preferences. Notably, unlike the references to the resources in many books, this one will actually be useful. One noteworthy exception is the case where the link helps with following up the subject of discussion (for instance, a webpage with Glycemic Index and Load in the corresponding section) – in such cases the link will be placed right in the book text.

In line with the idea of making this book your permanently working aid, the recipes in the Table of Contents have distinct font, making it easier to locate the one you need. The companion website http://timetraveldiet.com will have many more recipes as well as other related discussions, so I encourage you to follow it and join the discussion. Wherever black and white image wouldn't do a justice to a recipe, I have placed a reminder to go a gallery at the http://timetraveldiet.com/image-gallery/ where you will find full color photos illustrating the preparation technique or a completed dish.

Finally, many logical segments are followed by a quick summary of practical takeaways, making it easy to recall the most significant points.

FIRST PRONG:
MINUS SUGAR

Where Is It Hiding?

This, of course, is the first thing on your mind and on your doctor's lips when you start discussing your course of action after the diagnosis or discussing your weight loss. "Cut the sugar." Moreover, with all the newest revelations from all walks of life about the role excessive sugar intake plays in our well-being, I am reasonably confident this is not the first time you've heard it. So, I will assume that you are well aware of the menacing role that white sweet powder plays in our weight problems, cholesterol problems, blood sugar problems and whatever other problems come wrapped together in that grim package. With that, we can omit the "why sugar is bad" lecture and skip right to the heart of the matter: How to diminish its intake?

The practical problems that arise here are multifold. All sugars are not created equal, thus all sugars are not obvious to the casual observer. Some sugars are masqueraded as harmless by the manufacturers and sellers, which is not exactly true. Some sugars are hiding under different names or behind different stages of food digestion. Finally, as if detection problem wasn't enough, it can be downright difficult to break our long-cultivated habits and change our long-established tastes.

Let's untangle it all in this part, going over all things sugar-related and building the strategy of cutting out and replacing as much of it as possible and minimizing the harm from whatever's left. Let's start this topic with some theory. We are not going to make it overly heavy on science, and the understanding of these basics will be fairly useful in your everyday decisions.

Theory Behind Sugars

Before we dive into it, let's establish a rule of thumb for the things we eat: **The faster we digest it, the worse it is for our blood sugar levels**. The (simplified) mechanics behind this is: Quickly digested foods are easily and rapidly utilized for energy by your body – much more quickly than you can use this energy. Thus your blood sugar rises and your body uses insulin secretion to keep it down. Being a healthy person, you have a capacity to supress it successfully – for a time. If this cycle happens frequently and intensely, that capacity will diminish over time, leading to diabetes. Being diabetic, you are ill-equipped to combat such upsurges with insulin secretion. Post-meal blood sugar spikes cause inflammation, damage the lining of the blood vessels and negatively affect our body in many other ways.

Foods that take longer to digest don't lead to an immediate, sizeable inflow of energy, thus giving you a chance to gradually use the energy up.

To put it in practical terms, quickly digested foods include sugar (duh!), white bread, white rice, white potatoes, white flour pasta, candy bars or cakes (duh again). Add some fiber, minerals and vitamins, and you slow down digestion – think whole grain breads and pastas, oatmeal, bran cereal, some vegetables, some fruit. Add protein and fat, and you get the slowest digestion possible – we are talking beans, lentils, some dairy products, and meats. To find out where each food is on this scale, you can use a list of the Glycemic Load (GL) for various foods keeping this in mind:

- anything with a GL 10 or under is great
- anything with a GL between 11 and 19 is medium
- GL above 20 translates as diabetes multiplied by cardiac events (scary enough for you?)

The list is found here: http://www.health.harvard. edu/diseases-and-conditions/glycemic_index_and_ glycemic_load_for_100_foods

Having a quick look at the table, you can see what a measly 150 g of white rice does to your body – a GL at 43 is a murderer on your plate. Grapefruit at 3, on the contrary, is smiling at you from that fruit bowl on the counter.

Anything not on the list, just check with Google – there is little, if anything, that can't be found these days. Do keep in mind though: GL is good only as long as you can keep the portion size under control. See that Serving size column in the table? Watermelon sounds good with a GL at 4, IF you keep your limit to 120 grams (a hair over a 1/4 pound). So don't get encouraged by its low glycemic load and eat the whole thing.

Let's return for a second to that phrase: "giving you a chance to gradually use the energy up." This gives us a clue to one of the tricks we are going to incorporate in our weight loss and blood sugar taming program – **physical activity burns the sugar.** Let's combine it with the idea that adding fiber, protein and fat to the sugars and starches slows down the digestion, and the trick starts shaping up. Remember that for now, we will get back to it in the next section.

OK, back to digging into sugars. First of all, not all sugars are to be avoided at all costs. So, which sugars are bad and which are... well, good is probably not the right word at this stage, so let's say for now, not as bad? Let's make it simple: Pure sugars are bad as they go almost right into your bloodstream. Sugars with added fiber, protein and good fats are better as their digestion is not as rapid. In practice, it means that a spoon of sugar is bad (duh) while fruit is better – even if the fruit contains the same spoonful of sugar. By the same logic, whole fruit is better than a glass of juice from the same fruit. Not really news for you, I am sure – but hold on, this all is going to the foundation of our entire strategy of combatting our blood sugar spikes.

Are there sugars that we are told are better for us while they are not? Surely you are familiar with artificial sweeteners, sugar alcohols and other sugar substitutes. This topic can be highly confusing, with bewildering choices and perplexing terminology. One thing that is clear: Sugar substitutes are not the magic bullet that would allow you to satisfy your sweet tooth while avoiding all the negatives of sugar. They come with their own list of complications that make their consumption far from trouble-free. One particularly dangerous side is that they can create an impression that you can eat a lot of them. In fact, if you replace sugary foods by equal amounts of "sugar-free" where "free" means simply that a substitute is used in place of sugar, you are not likely to be much better. To be sure, some of them can help you a bit, but it involves more than simple substituting. Consider this from American Dietetic Association:

> "If you have diabetes, don't expect sugar substitutes to save the day. Think of mile-high piles of mashed potatoes or unlimited restaurant bread and tortilla chip baskets and you've probably already exceeded your carbohydrate intake. Although limited in number, studies generally show that simply using sugar substitutes alone without reducing carbohydrate from sugary, starchy foods (such as bread, rice or pasta) or fat (oils, high fat meat and dairy products) will probably not help control your blood sugar or blood fat levels."

Are there deceptive practices in naming and labeling things that we eat? Boy, are there ever! How many names do you think are being used to hide the sugar in plain sight from you? Over 60! Here is an alphabetic list. Notice how many of them do not have "sugar" or even "syrup" in their names:

Agave nectar, Barbados sugar, Barley malt, Barley malt syrup, Beet sugar, Blackstrap molasses, Brown sugar, Buttered syrup, Cane juice, Cane juice crystals, Cane sugar, Caramel, Carob syrup, Castor sugar, Coconut palm sugar, Coconut sugar, Confectioner's sugar, Corn sweetener, Corn syrup, Corn syrup solids, Crystalline fructose, Date sugar, Dehydrated cane juice, Demerara, Dextrin, Dextrose, Diatase, Diatastic malt, Ethyl maltol, Evaporated cane juice, Florida crystals, Free-flowing brown sugars, Fructose, Fruit juice, Fruit juice concentrate, Glucose, Glucose solids, Golden sugar, Golden syrup, Grape sugar, HFCS (High-Fructose Corn Syrup), Honey, Icing sugar, Invert sugar, Malt syrup, Maltodextrin, Maltol, Maltose, Mannose, Maple syrup, Molasses, Muscovado, Palm sugar, Panela, Panocha, Powdered sugar, Raw sugar, Refiner's syrup, Rice syrup, Saccharose, Sorghum Syrup, Sucanat, Sucrose, Sugar (granulated), Sweet Sorghum Syrup, Treacle, Turbinado, Yellow sugar.

Some names are even naturally deceptive. Think fructose is better for you because it's fruity-sounding? Think again – as an added sugar it's even more harmful for you than your garden variety glucose.

Think you are a sophisticated label reader and know that the closer the ingredient is to the beginning the more there is in the product? Think again: Manufacturers break down sugar content by several names, so they move to the seventh or eighth place in the list, and you feel you can shrug it off. Meanwhile, added together they would have moved sugar to the beginning of the list! There, Muscovado, Panocha, Mannose and Treacle conspire to kill you per Diatase orders and under Turbinado's guidance, and you don't even know what they all are.

Bottom line is: While whole foods do contain some natural sugars together with fiber, nutrients and various beneficial compounds, packaged and processed foods are laced with added sugar that greatly exceeds our healthy intake limits and that is very difficult to spot, let alone avoid. Even foods generally considered healthy, like yogurt, can and often do have added sugar in them. Why, you ask? The answer is easy. In the words of Robert Lustig, M.D., professor of pediatrics in the division of endocrinology at the University of California, *"You could make dog poop taste good with enough sugar, and the food industry does."* It's also addictive, which means you are going to want and eat more.

Now that we are more aware of the numerous faces of sugar, are we armed with enough knowledge to move to the practical steps? Not yet, there is one more thing to deal with before we do. It is an issue of the foods that are not sugars per se but are so close to them in the digestion chain that the practical difference is too insignificant, so they are almost as hazardous for us. We are back to those simple carbohydrates that we mentioned earlier – those that get broken down to sugars so easily and so fast that their effect is just as harmful. Those are starchy foods with low to no fiber content: White breads, cereals, potatoes, pastas, and rice, highly processed, highly refined, finely milled. When we say "fast break down to sugars," just how fast is fast? Here is an approximate breakdown:

- Juice is almost always immediately turned to sugar.
- Simple carbs become sugar anywhere from 5 minutes to 30-60 minutes after eating.
- The higher the fiber and solids content (think veggies/whole grains/legumes), the slower the carbs turn to sugar, dragging the process up to 2 hours.
- Protein begins breaking down into sugar about 2 hours after eating.
- Fat can take up to 3-4 hours.

Just one last comment before we go into the practical part. While we have stated that starches are generally a poor choice as they are just one step removed from sugars, there is one specific and intriguing way to deal with them that deserves a separate segment. We will get to it in the Resistant Starches section.

Sugary Drinks

Hopefully, you are one of those folks who don't have this addiction, and pop drinks are not a part of your daily consumption. If so, congratulations, and you can just surf through this section to glean some healthy and tasty drink ideas that might come in handy. If you do have this problem, this is where you start; make this your very first step in your journey.

Let's also devise a simple test of whether or not your taste buds lose their sensitivity to sugar, thus demanding more and more of it to feel satisfied. Find a large, ripe, juicy Granny Smith apple and take a good bite. Is it sweet enough or do you perceive it as a cardboard imitation, with not much taste to it? If the latter is true, in all likelihood your sensitivity to sugar has been dulled.

Some things bringing excessive sugar into our bodies need to be cut out – those steps are simple (not necessarily easy, but simple). Some require a more complicated approach – replacing them with other foods or components in the food we make. Such replacements naturally necessitate trying new recipes, tweaking old ones, adjusting our routines and sometimes tastes. Let's start with the simple things; they are our natural beginning point and the results are immediately noticeable.

The most obvious sugars we consume are in our drinks. Soda drinks; tea or coffee with added sugar;

fancy Frappuccinos, where the blend of strawberries and cream with white chocolate sauce is topped with whipped cream and a sprinkle of chocolate; caramelized honey latte topped with steamed milk. You get the idea. I won't list all of the sugar content in those; suffice it to say that a **single** 12 oz. (355 ml) can of Coca Cola already exceeds your entire recommended daily intake of added sugar. Oh, and so does a "venti-sized" Frappuccino which, with all of the toppings easily gets you about 400 calories (a small meal) in a very sneaky manner – meaning that you are going to feel hungry much faster than after consuming a similar number of calories with actual food.

Let's be honest about these drinks. Other than an occasional treat, they simply have to be dropped altogether from your diet. There is no sugar-coating this: they have no place in a healthy nutrition regimen. They also constitute a rare exception to the concept of returning to our diet upon completion of the weight loss program; I can't in good conscience consider them a part of a sensible nutrition regimen.

But if you are used to drinking them, how do you go about getting rid of them? Here is one thing that is going to help you. In an elegantly paradoxical way, this is that same thing that makes added sugar so dangerous for us. Here are two things that sugar does to us:

1   It retrains our taste buds so that we like sweet things, identify "tasty" with "sweet" and at the same time lose our sensitivity to the sweetness; it dulls our taste receptors and that leads us to seek out more and more sugar content.

2 It creates a sugar rush followed by a crash, which makes us crave more sugary foods. The impact on our brain is not unlike the addiction created by drugs; it feeds into ever-increasing dissatisfaction with current levels of sugar consumption and makes us seek more.

Sounds quite gloomy, doesn't it? Where is the silver lining in this? Here it is: This spiral that supports consumption increase works in the same way in the opposite direction, once you break its momentum. In practical terms it means that the hardest part is to begin phasing out sugary drinks; once the process takes root it becomes easier and easier, accelerating day by day and quickly taking you to a state where you can't even taste that soda because it's so over-sweetened.

This is a very important moment that I would like to stop and analyze here, because we are going to encounter this in many ways and respects down the road. When we experience discomfort, unpleasant sensations, lack of certain foods or a particular taste, we expect this unpleasantness to stay, probably increase until becoming unbearable. This expectation by itself makes us more likely to cease the action that caused discomfort. In other words, it's fear of the pain that makes us quit, and not the actual pain. The reality, however, is different. Our body adjusts quickly to doing healthy things and the discomfort goes away instead of increasing. If you do not give up at the first strong craving or first sharp pang of hunger, it doesn't increase – it goes away. It returns now and then, in waves – and each new episode is weaker and weaker, easier and easier to deal with. It's almost as if our body sends these signals of distress to demand something, but if the signal doesn't get met with the subject of demand, body stops begging. Being a creature of habit, our body wants to maintain a routine; it protests when the routine is broken, but if there is no return to it, it gets used to a new routine and enjoys it just as faithfully. It's trainable; we just need to train it instead of rewarding its protest by meeting its demands. The ultimate purpose of this training is not merely to teach our body to stop demanding harmful things. It's also to train it to ask for the good things, so we start enjoying eating and practicing them. Then, and only then, our life becomes healthy and happy; instead of making a constant effort to eat right and live right, we do it naturally and enjoy it.

We will encounter and utilize this phenomenon many times in our journey. It will also play a major role in our final blow to our weight problem and help us lose excess fat.

In light of all that, let's work out this view on everything we do: this is retraining. Many of our harmful habits are not naturally ingrained; they are learned. Retraining our body, retraining our habits and reactions, retraining our entire mindset with the purpose of creating a new set of routines and practices where we do not have to force ourselves to do what's good for us – our entire way of life makes it natural and enjoyable.

Think back to any time when you learned to do something new. It usually went through the same sequence, starting with effort, forcing yourself to do something difficult at first, becoming easier and easier with practice until it became easy and effortless. Learning to drive for instance? Riding a bike? Any hobby you enjoy? Pick any example of any activity at which you became good and return mentally to the times when you practiced doing it. This is the same sequence you are going to go through once again. Such a view will help us overcome the first hurdle, with our sight set firmly on the goal.

Finally, let's touch on your first motivation to sever that leash holding you in sugar slavery. Sure, there is a desire to become slimmer and healthier; but when it comes to dropping those sugary drinks, add one more thought. It IS slavery, and your captors want you to stay dumb, happy, oblivious and to consume more of their product. If that doesn't make you feel annoyed, you are going to remain their ideal captive – one that won't leave his prison even when the door is unlocked and unguarded. That's not how I see myself and, I am sure, neither do you. The determination to become a master of your own well-being should become your incentive on this first step. Gratification from success will help immensely after that, giving you a great sense of being in control; reversing the spiral of addiction will make each next step easier.

Once the decision is made, let's start cutting down on the sugar portions. At some point I used to put 4 teaspoons of sugar in my tea. If I tried to drink it with no sugar at all, it would taste like liquid cardboard. There is no point in trying to shock your body by cutting its drug of choice at once; we don't want it to start protesting, we want it to start the process of retraining. So, instead of heroic attempts to quit cold turkey, let's cut the intake gradually. Several days of 3 teaspoons instead of 4, and it becomes the new norm; move to 2 and give it a few days more. When you do it this way, it causes no real problems. All you have to endure is the first day or two, then your taste buds stop noticing the change. That process of the reverse spiral we mentioned earlier starts working. Next, when you come to no sugar at all, instead of ignoring absence of taste, start focusing on the taste of the tea or coffee itself. If it's a tea, make sure it's an interesting one, with good flavor – say, a mix with a peach flavor, rose petals or whatever else you like. If it's a coffee, get a good brand with deep rich flavor. You see, sugar masks any flavor of the original drink. You can't taste it anymore; sugar simply replaces the original taste – in the same way ketchup buries any underlying taste so you can't sense anything but the ketchup itself. Thus, it makes perfect sense to have a pleasant and interesting flavor to focus on and to give yourself a chance to taste that flavor. Evicting sugar from your drinks, you suddenly discover the whole world of new tastes previously hidden from you.

While we are talking about coffee, try this: get a square of a good dark chocolate and slowly, enjoying every morsel, eat it before the first sip of your strong black coffee. You will be amazed by how they work together to create a deep, combined taste and create a whole new appreciation for good coffee. No milk or cream is needed – in fact, they kill the native taste of coffee.

Now that you can feel the taste of the tea and coffee, make a point to discover new great flavors. Look for loose teas of course, not the tea bags. Visit specialized tea stores, desirably small locally owned ones and not the large chains. Smell the teas that intrigue you. Ask for the sample size bags of those that impress you with their scent. Try different coffee brands. You will soon have a few kinds you like for different seasons, occasions and times of the day. Their taste will become new addition to your food delights. However difficult it might be for you to believe it prior retraining, a few weeks later you won't even be able to drink them with sugar. You also won't understand how you could like them with sugar earlier. People still doing that are going to make you wonder why they would eliminate the specific taste of the very drink they consume. It's almost as if you needed sugar to mask a taste of a bad drink – but then again, why would you want to have a bad drink? Why not go for a good drink instead and enjoy its own taste?

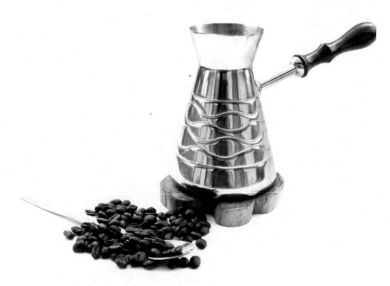

JEZVA, TURKISH COFFEE POT

To give you ideas to start with, some of our favorite teas are Ice Wine, Black Currant, Mango, Plum, Peach (all organic, you don't want chemical taste imitations). The list changes now and then, as we get to try new ones or as our favorite vendor says "Got a new mix for you guys to taste." Try black, green, white, oolong, rooibos. They are all different, and many are fabulous.

As far as coffee concerned, we prefer a medium roast Colombian Arabica, in a form of whole beans which we grind ourselves every day in portions enough for one brew. Our preferred method of brewing is traditional Turkish coffee pot called jezva. This is strong coffee, but once you tried it...

Don't think you need to emulate our preferences. Whatever you enjoy is great. Just make sure that you stay curious and open to try new kinds – that guarantees that you don't get tired.

Now is a good time to introduce two more hot drinks that will add variety and bring numerous health benefits. One is **ROASTED CHICORY ROOT**, a caffeine free coffee alternative that is even somewhat close to the taste of coffee – rich and deep, somewhat bitter. It has anti-inflammation properties, is full of antioxidants, and increases bile production helping metabolize fats. Most importantly, it contains inulin – a prebiotic, indigestible fiber (we will get more familiar with this concept later in this part) which helps our digestion and keeps down blood sugar level. It's sold in granules which you can steep for 8-10 minutes in a cup of boiled water using a tea strainer, 1 tablespoon per cup. It can also benefit from a lemon wedge added to a cup – experiment with variations to find your preferred taste.

Another is **CINNAMON**, commonly known for many health benefits and among them – to help regulate blood sugar. This spice also combines easily with many additional ingredients, thus leaving plenty of room for experiments and variety of tastes. Try lemon, ginger, turmeric, minced apple, cloves, mint, orange zest or any combination of those. You can use cinnamon sticks, about 3 inches long per a cup of hot water. Let the stick sit in the boiled water for a while if you want it to release more of its components and produce a deeper taste. You may want to do that in advance and then reheat the drink. Alternatively, you can use ground cinnamon. A teaspoon per cup of boiled water steeped for 8-10 minutes will do the trick.

Speaking of soda drinks, resist the temptation to continue drinking their diet versions. Replacing one poison with another won't help you much. For the details about this particular kind of poison, refer to the Resources section with the list of studies. Our idea is to stop poisoning ourselves. To accomplish that, if you do need some interesting flavor instead of a pop drink, do some experimenting with the following additives to your water:

- lemon slices;
- cucumber slices;
- vanilla beans or extract;
- citrus zest;
- cocoa;
- cinnamon;
- nutmeg;
- mint;
- ginger.

Needless to say, there are endless combinations of these. Make it fun experimenting to find your flavor, or even a few. Oh, and while we are on it: disabuse yourself of any possible delusions about store-bought smoothies, bottled ice-teas, energy drinks, vitamin-enriched waters and whatever else is being industriously pushed on us to sell us more sugar.

Now, what do you do if it's not just the taste but sweetness of the soda drinks that is so irresistible and you just can't give that up? If your idea of a replacement is fruit juices, forget that – they contain all the sugar but little to no fiber of an actual fruit. Your bridge can be one of these steps, or all of them simultaneously:

- start diluting your soda with water to wean yourself off that sugar influx gradually;
- eat some fruit with your unsweetened drink, to compensate the lost sweetness. This way you still get some sugar, but it's accompanied with fiber and nutrition, thus slowing down the blood sugar spike and not being just empty calories. Strawberries with their very low glycemic load are an excellent choice;
- eat a portion of protein with your drink. This will further supress blood sugar spikes, reducing food cravings and minimizing harm. Several almonds or walnuts will do, just as some cold cuts with leafy veggies; it's as simple as that.
- make sure that you get physically active after your drink. Take a quick walk, do some push-ups and squats; burn that excessive energy not letting it turn into stored form.

In the last three tips you no doubt can recognize the application of the principles we described in the theory section. Notice that we are talking about eating whole fruit or berries here, not squeezing them in your water – this way you do get the benefit of fiber. Remember the trick we mentioned a few pages earlier, combining rapidly-digested food with slowly-digested? Here is how to implement it, and in more instances than just with drinks. When at any point in your undertaking you do want something sweet, there is no point in completely denying yourself that marvellous pastry or a piece of a fabulous cake. We do not intend to make our life a glum string of days filled with sullen rejection of all the enjoyable things. Instead, we want to relish them while keeping the harmful aspects at bay. Thus, knowing the exact mechanics of how those sweets can harm us, we consume them in a smart way. We make sure that **they are accompanied by fiber and protein and scheduled around the time of physical activity**. Addition of healthy food will slow down the digestion, while activity will help to burn the excess of energy before it goes into storage. Plan to have your sweet treat before you go for a walk or ride a stationary bike with a good book in hand and have that treat together with an added portion of slowly digested food.

Speaking of tricks, let me throw another one your way. It's ages-old and undeservedly abandoned in favor of store-bought sweets. Take that Granny Smith, wrap it in foil and put it in the counter-top oven for 15 min (usual oven or barbeque will do just as well). Exact time depends on how firm it is and how mushy you want it to become, so you may want to experiment a bit to find which variation you like the best. Heated up and somewhat mushy, it becomes a real treat, a valid dessert. Want to add a curious taste? Sprinkle it with cinnamon. Add some crushed walnut or sunflower seeds for crunchiness and protein. Got other ideas how to tweak it? Go for it; create your own dessert out of the most common fruit on earth. Further in the book we will introduce a few more healthy and unconventional dessert ideas, but this one requires nothing but willingness to try, so why not add it to your arsenal right now.

Let's at this point repeat the "apple test" here, to evaluate how your retraining process takes root. See any changes? You should start enjoying it much more, noticing its natural sweetness and distinctive taste. That's your taste buds becoming more sensitive to sugar. At this point some of the formerly enjoyed over-sweetened treats start tasting unbearably and unpleasantly sweet.

What you might be missing when cutting out soda drinks is their pleasant fizziness. At first, using carbonated water can help. Further in this book we will introduce a home-made probiotic drink called kombucha. If you are impatient to experience its amazing (and variable) taste and numerous health benefits, feel free to jump to that section. There is no rigid sequence in this, you can mix and match as many elements of this whole endeavour as you please.

All the steps listed should not take you longer than a few weeks to wean yourself off sugary drinks. Hopefully, by this time not only have you successfully cut sugary drinks out of your life, but also got a taste of just how exciting this journey can be. You might also find out that in the middle of this gradual elimination of sugar in your drinks you are suddenly ready to drop it to zero at once; try to listen to yourself and stay sensitive to your body's reactions, to catch the moment when addiction takes its claws off you.

At this point you should be noticing the first benefits of your efforts. Have you ever experienced sleepiness after a meal? This should diminish noticeably. The same goes for hunger spikes, chaotic food cravings at odd times. Your hunger bouts should decrease and even out through the day. And of course, you will notice the first changes on your bathroom scales. And those are only external changes. Inflammation in your blood vessels calming down, cholesterol normalization, stomach lining healing – all this slowly and quietly starts happening under the hood, to manifest themselves later in longer years of better health.

Here is good news: this was probably the most difficult step! If you have accomplished it, you will be able to walk the rest of the path. More so, everything you are going to do next will be more and more fascinating and encouraging. For now, congratulations: this was your first step to liberation. You didn't just taste the sugarless drinks – you tasted freedom from an enslaving sugar addiction.

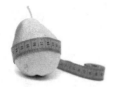

PRACTICAL TAKEAWAY: QUICK SUMMARY

- Rapidly digested foods turn into sugar quickly in our digestive system; those are mostly simple carbohydrates.

- Adding fiber, protein and fat slows down their digestion and gives us time to burn the sugar off. Planning sweet foods so they are followed by physical activity supresses their harmful effects.

- Processed foods are often full of sugars disguised under different names.

- Our taste buds lose sensitivity to sugar and demand more of it; we learn to identify sweet with tasty. Both processes are reversible. Our body can be trained to break the slavery of sugary foods.

- Simple yet interesting drinks can replace pop drinks and sugary hot drinks easily. Use fruit and berry to sweeten them naturally. Use chicory and cinnamon hot drinks to reap additional health benefits.

Replacing Starchy Foods

As you remember, our next stop in the sugar hierarchy is starches – white bread, white rice, pasta, potato. These are the foods that are so close to sugar that they break down to sugars in a very short time, causing very similar consequences. Being a strong heroic type and excluding them outright is too extreme an approach. We don't want that. Instead, we want joy with no punishment. This is possible with substitutes that come closer (an in some cases even better!) and with some interesting tweaks which we will discuss in the next section.

PASTA

Let's look at those substitutes. I would like to start with pasta, and there is a good reason for that. One of my favorite dishes for many years was, and remains, seafood pasta made on an olive oil base. One thing that used to upset me about it was that I could have it only rarely. Can we replace the usual pasta with something better, yet just as tasty? I am not talking here about the whole wheat or whole grain variations; while those are superior to their white refined siblings, we can do even better. Let's see. Usual white pasta nutrition facts, per 50 g of dry product:

- Carbohydrates: 37.3g

- Fiber: 1.6g
- Protein: 6.5g

White pasta's whole wheat brother fares a tad better, most of improvement being in fiber:

- Carbohydrates: 37.5g
- Fiber: 4.2g
- Protein: 7.3

We can do much better though. There is pasta with merely 15g of carbs, of which a whopping 11g is fiber and with 22g of protein. Oh, and it tastes amazing, and has this great firm to the bite texture that Italians call al dente. In case you haven't tried that yet, I believe you are in for a surprise. I am talking about **BLACK BEAN SPAGHETTI** – black beans and water, nothing else. Here is how it looks dry:

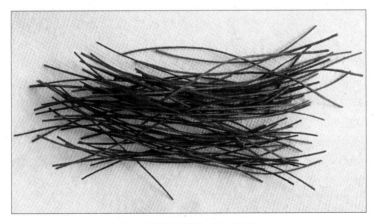

BLACK BEAN PASTA, DRY

7 minutes in boiling water, and you are there – just mix it with whatever you like in your pasta. But, since I mentioned my favorite seafood pasta, this is a good place to share the recipe.

You will need a mix of seafood goodies – mussels, shrimp, calamari, scallops and whatever else they put in those bags with seafood medley. Purchase such a medley or put together your own of your favorite sea creatures. Thaw them if they are frozen and press them a bit to squeeze out the water. Cook your pasta according to the (shamefully uncomplicated) instructions on the package. Grab a wok, pour some olive oil on the bottom, press a few garlic cloves and drop them in the oil. Take the oil to a gentle boil – when you see it bubbling and smell the garlic, turn the heat down to medium. Drop the seafood medley in the oil and mix it with wooden spoons so that your creatures get infused with oil and garlic. If you have cooked shrimp and mussels in the mix, reserve them for now lest they get overcooked. Squid and scallop don't require much; usually they are ready within 5-7 minutes simmered gently. Bite the squid to determine readiness – when you can bite through it, it's ready. Now add shrimp and mussels and cook for 1-2 min more. Add the pasta and continue mixing the whole combination blending together all the components and making sure the pasta gets soaked in the liquid. As you mix, add salt, pepper and your favorite herbs to taste – oregano and parsley usually work well.

Please see a gallery at the http://timetraveldiet.comimage-gallery/ for the full color photo illustrating Seafood pasta, served.

There you go – my favorite pasta as often as I want, full of protein and fiber, wheat-free, starch-free, gluten-free and guilt-free! I am sure you will have no problem coming up with endless variations with this product, from pastas to soups.

Speaking of pasta substitutes, there is more to try. There is high protein chickpea rotini, black beans rotini, high in fiber quinoa pasta, buckwheat-based soba and more. Have fun experimenting and enjoy new tastes.

Please see a gallery at the http://timetraveldiet.com/image-gallery/ for the full color photo illustrating wheat free pastas.

POTATO

Meanwhile, we made our first step replacing starches in our diet with their healthier brethren. Let's make another. Who doesn't like **FRIES** ? I see no raised hands. Mine stays on the table as well. I love them... and don't eat them. As tasty as they are, my body tells me they are not good for me. I feel heavy and sleepy after eating them and my blood sugar shoots up like clockwork. The substitute I offer has none of those side effects.

Fair warning: this one may seem a bit puzzling. The thing is, if you go purely with a side-by-side comparison per nutrition data websites, you won't see much benefit to the substitute I suggest to try. While there are some mentions of the microelements that lower inflammation factors, the research confirming that is beyond my, and probably your, capabilities. One factor, however, is easy to find and evaluate, and this is probably what explains the effect: while potatoes have a high glycemic index of 85, the replacement we discuss has a nice low 46. The glycemic load is almost twice as low. That alone can account for the difference. In any case, if you ever noticed that potato fries make you feel heavy, tired, sleepy, and cause some tummy aches, just try this idea once and see if you notice any difference. If this proves true for you as it did for me, you have your way to have those delicious fries with all the benefits of tubers' nutrients but without the penalty.

The substitute we are talking about is cassava, also known as yuca root. Sometimes it's mislabeled in the stores as yucca root, which is actually a different plant altogether. To avoid the confusion, make sure that it looks like the image in a gallery shows.

Please see a gallery at the http://timetraveldiet.com/image-gallery/ for the full color photo illustrating Yuca root, a.k.a. cassava

To prepare it, trim off both tapered ends and cut the root in half. Remove and discard the skin with your knife – it's hard and inedible. Cut the root lengthwise in half, and again in half to have four quarters. Now remove and discard the woody core from the inner corner of each quarter – it looks like a long stringy thread. Cut the flesh in the shape and size of the fries. Drop your fries in cold water and let them stay there for 10-15 minutes to remove some starch (if you can prepare them in advance, do that and soak them for a few hours to remove even more). You will see white powder in the water making it milky – that's starch you want to decrease in your fries. By the way, use the same trick if you prepare standard issue potatoes. Discard the water.

Now for cooking itself. Pour the fresh water in again and heat it to a boil on the stovetop. Let the fries boil for 15 minutes and poke them with a fork. You want them to become soft so the fork can pierce them; anywhere from 15 to 25 minutes depending on the size of your fries should be enough. Meanwhile preheat your oven to 450F. Strain the water (you will see that it became milky again, which indicates more starch removed). Rinse the fries with cold water. Drizzle with olive oil, garlic, coarse salt, pepper and/or whatever else you like with your fries – some prefer chili powder, onion flakes, sundried tomato, rosemary etc. Place them on the baking sheet covered with foil, as close to one layer as possible. Put the sheet in the oven and bake for 15 minutes. Flip the fries and return them to oven for another 15 min. If you want a crispier look and feel, try the broiler for a few minutes. All the times are approximate as the size to which you cut them varies. Just experiment a bit to get the texture you like. Eat them with your favorite barbeque sauce (go easy on those though, they are full of sugar!) or without; they reheat well if you make too much for one sitting. Keep in mind that cassava's calorie count is higher than potato's, so you get your fill with less of it.

While we discuss the replacement for the potato, you may wonder why we limit this to fries when there is also such a delicious thing as **MASHED POTATOES.** Sure enough, while there is a cauliflower as a widely known substitute for potato, cassava works for this just as well if not better. Cut it in thick chunks. Boil it about 20-25 minutes, or until soft when tested with a fork. Keep in mind that you may have to experiment a bit with this, since over-boiled cassava tends to have somewhat gelatinous texture and result in too runny final dish. Here is my preferred version of it:

- 2 pounds yuca root
- 1 head of roasted garlic
- 4 Tbsp butter
- 1 cup buttermilk
- salt and pepper to taste

While the garlic is being roasted, peel and cut cassava to small cubes. Boil it and drain off the water. Then add buttermilk, butter and garlic and mash it with a wooden spoon or a potato masher. Season and serve.

Make any variations to match the way you like mashed potato – there are so many versions of it, with milk, half-and-half, sour cream, vinegar, bacon, nutmeg, herbs and whatnot that I wouldn't even try to list them all. You have your base covered by cassava – now get inspired and create the best mashed potato-less potato your family ever tried!

Speaking of potatoes, we can't omit **PANCAKES** (or their ever-popular variation, **latkes**). With all the known variations, the base of the recipe is usually grated potato and all-purpose flour. In the spirit of our replacement strategy, we substitute the grated cassava for potato and tapioca flour for an all-purpose one. In case you wonder what tapioca flour is, it's made from this same cassava – perfect replacement for the all-purpose flour, wheat-, grain-, dairy-, gluten- and (almost) sugar-free. If you have tapioca starch in the stores around you, don't worry, it's the same thing. We will touch on other substitutes after the recipe.

Basic recipe (actually, it's so basic that I hesitate to cite here; I could just as well write simply "make a pancake"): boil yuca as described above. Squeeze it to separate and drain as much liquid as you can. Draining out the moisture is an important step ensuring crisp pancakes. Add tapioca flour and mix well. Heat a non-stick skillet over medium-high heat, and add 1 teaspoon vegetable oil (I prefer grapeseed oil for that). When very hot, add batter and season to taste with salt and pepper. Use a spatula to press the batter into a flat, round shape. Reduce heat to medium, and cook until golden-brown, 5 to 7 minutes. Flip pancake, add the teaspoon of oil around the edges of the pancake and season again with salt and pepper. Continue cooking until golden-brown and crisp on both sides, 5 to 7 minutes more. Done.

If you want to get a bit fancier:

- 2 cups of yuca root
- 1 egg
- 1 yellow onion
- 2 Tbsp tapioca flour
- salt and pepper to taste
- vegetable oil for frying (to repeat, grapeseed oil is my preference)

Boil yucca root as described above and squeeze it to separate and drain as much liquid as you can. Chop the onion finely and squeeze out the water as well. Beat the egg lightly with salt and pepper. Mix the egg, onion and flour with yuca root, making sure that you just mix but not whip it. Heat ¼ inch oil in a skillet over medium-high heat. Drop three or four mounds of the batter into hot oil to make half-inch thick pancakes; press to flatten if needed. Fry until they turn golden-brown, about 3 min per side. Serve with sour cream.

For variations, try to add garlic, parmesan cheese, farmer cheese, cayenne pepper... you got the idea, there is nothing to limit your creativity here. Now, want to change the taste profile and add some protein to your pancakes? Try chickpeas flour instead of tapioca. Or buckwheat flour. See if it works for you, and remember these two for now, they will play a large role in our diet preferences just a few pages down.

Before we move further, let's mention another widely known and commonly used substitute for potato. I am talking about sweet potato of course. While it's a valid replacement, let's state two important points about it. First, you need to eat it with the skin. Comparing the glycemic response to a peeled sweet potato and one with skin shows a drastic difference – so much so that there were even attempts to create a blood sugar lowering supplement from the skin alone. Take a look at the illustration from *Glycemic Index of Sweet Potato as Affected by Cooking Methods*, published in The Open Nutrition Journal, 2012, 6, 1-11. It needs to be viewed in color, so I am going to refer you to the online gallery. You can see at 30 min after consumption glucose from the flesh alone is 6 times (!) greater than from the whole thing:

Please see a gallery at the http://timetraveldiet.com/image-gallery/ for the full color photo illustrating sweet potato glucose response.

Another point: for some reason there are way more recipes for a sweet potato with sugar or marshmallows than savoury ones. Dismiss those sweetened versions. Make it with olive oil or butter, salt, garlic, pepper and herbs, mix it with vegetables. In other words, treat it as a savoury side dish and not as a dessert.

RICE

Having successfully replaced pasta and potatoes, we need to cover another staple starchy food – rice. I don't have to tell you that white rice is not really a good food for our case. 1 cup has 205 calories, 45 g carbs, a measly 1 g. of fiber, 4 g. of protein – but worst of all, its glycemic index is 73 (89 and higher yet for some variations) and the glycemic load is 43. Reading those numbers alone can send your blood sugar through the roof. Sure, there is brown rice, and you most likely are familiar with its benefits. It's about the same in calories and carbs, but it has 4 times as much fiber and its glycemic load stands at 16, with the index being 63. Better, right? We can do better yet though.

Enter the somewhat confusing name: parboiled rice. Confusing, because it sounds very close to pre-boiled or pre-cooked rice, which is what many mistake it for. No rice is worse for you that a pre-boiled (also known as minute or instant) rice. Parboiled though is a whole different animal. Not only its glycemic load is lower yet, merely 14, but its glycemic index is just 38! Also, the somewhat unusual preparation process allows it to preserve a higher content of vitamins than any of its brethren. You may also find parboiled rice under the name "converted" – it's the same process and the same product.

Since it has lower fiber content than brown rice, you will do well using it in recipes and combinations that add legumes or leafy vegetables.

Speaking of recipes, my favorite for rice is pilaf or plov. There are endless versions of this amazing dish. Most of them combine rice with various kinds of meat and vegetable, adding protein, fat and fiber. The dish itself is a bit complicated, so in keeping with the spirit of simplicity in this book I won't recite the recipe here; just search for the pilaf with meat of your preference (or a vegetarian version) and you will come up with many ways to cook it. Those that use onion and carrot for vegetable addition and cumin in spices will be closer to the original recipes.

Having discussed several replacements for the starchy foods, I have another step in mind, and it's really good one. We can take our quest to make starches less of a foe and more of a friend even further. Going back to par-boiled rice, there is one important detail about it. You may have asked yourself: with such low fiber content, what is the source of its delightfully low glycemic index? How can it be? The answer triggers whole new area of knowledge, opening wonderful opportunities to better nourishment. It deserves its own section. Read on.

Resistant Starches

Starch is bad for our blood sugar and our waist. We know this from both theory and practice. Theory tells us that starch is merely one step above sugar, and breaks down to sugar in no time. Practice confirms that – diets rich in white bread, potato and white rice expand our midline like no other. Yet there is one type of starch that is good for our health, our blood sugar and our figure. That's resistant starch.

What on earth is resistant starch you ask? Actually, the name is quite self-explanatory. It resists digestion. It doesn't get broken down by the enzymes in our small intestine; instead, it travels into large intestine where it becomes a prebiotic – food for our gut bacteria (the good kind; we will speak more of it in the Second Prong, for now just know that this is the kind of bacteria that we want to nourish). In doing so, resistant starch combines the benefit of both soluble and insoluble fiber.

The positive effect of consuming resistant starches is difficult to overestimate. They help us burn fat, boost metabolism, increase insulin sensitivity, lower fasting blood sugar and supress the glycemic response. They contribute to digestive health, improve sleep and decrease inflammation in the gut and other tissues. They improve blood lipid profile (cholesterol!) and promote colonic health. To throw some science into the mix, during their fermentation in the large intestine, our body produces short chain fatty acids, of which butyrate is of particular importance. Butyrate is needed for our digestive system to function properly, positively influences our immune system and participates in countless processes necessary for our overall health. There are more benefits to resistant starches being discovered every day (it's a relatively new field, mostly appearing in the 1980s and developing ever since), but everything listed should be convincing enough for us to include them in our diet.

Now, what does it all have to do with that parboiled rice and its intriguingly low glycemic index? Everything; the process of its preparation includes something called retrogradation. The starch in uncooked rice or potato is indigestible. When we cook it, however, it turns fully digestible – and becomes that same foe we defined before, the usual starch that we try to avoid. In the process of preparing parboiled rice, the rice is cooled following a temperature treatment (steaming), some of the starch turns back into its resistant form, and stays that way, even during cooking or reheating. That's the source of this kind of rice's low glycemic index.

But wait... if cooling these starches off after a temperature treatment triggers retrogradation and turns some of the starch into desirable form, what about cooked potato? Yup! Make your usual potato dish, let it cool and put it in the fridge overnight. Tomorrow you will have a much healthier (or less harmful, if you prefer) mashed potato or fries. The best thing about it is, you won't have to eat it cold – reheating doesn't turn resistant starch back into digestible.

(As a bonus idea: corn on the cob? Instead of cooking one every day while they are in season, make more than you need, enjoy one hot, and refrigerate the rest. They will be as delicious tomorrow either cold or hot, and you will reap the benefits of retrogradation).

Let's throw a bit of science-speak here, so this process doesn't sound like a miracle:

EFFECT OF RETROGRADATION
ON STARCH DIGESTIBILITY

Native starch is digested slowly by enzymes due to the highly ordered molecular structure in intact granules. Processing or cooking disrupts the ordered structure of granular starch, resulting in the increased susceptibility of starch to enzymatic digestion (Wang and Copeland 2013). Subsequent cooling and storage leads to retrogradation, in which starch regains an ordered structure that is more resistant to enzymatic digestion (Eerlingen and others 1994; Cui and Oates 1997; Chung and others 2006; Zhou and Lim 2012).[*]

Notice how recent many of these studies are. If you haven't heard of this before, no wonder: We are dealing with cutting edge research here (I consider that rather unfortunate since the studies in such cases tend to be scant and preliminary, and the methods are inconsistent). Even though there is a work titled "Digestibility of

---

[*]   *Starch Retrogradation: A Comprehensive Review* by Shujun Wang, Caili Li, Les Copeland, Qing Niu, and Shuo Wang, 2015

starch of different sorts as affected by cooking" by Edna D. Day discussing these very matters published in 1908(!), the importance of it has been realized relatively recently, and the field of research has grown rapidly ever since. In fact, in 1998 the Joint Food and Agricultural Organization of the United Nations/World Health Organization Expert Consultation on Human Nutrition concluded that resistant starch is *"...one of the major developments in our understanding of the importance of carbohydrates for health in the past twenty years."*

As far as scientific confirmation of all the findings specific to diabetes, I'll quote the Nutrition Bulletin Volume 30, from March 2005, titled Health properties of resistant starch by A. P. Nugent:

> *"Most studies in humans have focused on postprandial glycaemic and/or insulinaemic responses and have varied in quality (see below). There is a lack of consensus regarding the precise effects of RS on insulin and glucose responses: 15 studies have reported an improvement in these measures following the consumption of a RS-rich test-meal, while 10 have showed no, or a physiologically irrelevant effect. It is noteworthy that, to date, there are no reports of RS worsening insulin and glucose responses."*

Back to practice. Two additional pieces of information that have practical applications for us:

1 Cooling these starches off for about six hours, down to 39 degrees F, produces most of

retrogradation; after that, the process slows down in a significant way. Therefore, cooling these foods overnight in the fridge is sufficient to acquire the desired effect.

2 Re-warming these foods and subsequently cooling them back down again noticeably increases the resistance starch content even further. Therefore, cook a few days' worth and when reheating a portion for a meal, let the rest warm up to room temperature before putting it back in the fridge. You will reap the increased benefits as you work your way through that pilaf or mashed potato.

How much of the starch content turns into resistant form? According to the Potato Nutrition Handbook published by The United States Potato Board, baked potato has up to 1g of RS per 100g, while cooked and cooled has 3.2g. That's a significant increase, especially considering that we have a two-pronged effect: Reduction of the digestible starch and turning it into fiber. However, that's far from turning ALL of it – there is still about 20g of starch in a cooked potato, so we still have a significant portion of digestible form left. Thus, let's put it in perspective: the trick we discussed cuts down on the harmful effects of starchy foods, but doesn't eliminate those effects in full.

This naturally takes us to the next question. Since resistant starches are so beneficial for us, how do we ensure proper daily intake? The general recommendation is 30-40g a day. Some improvements seem to take place at as little as 10g a day and above 50-60g there is no apparent additional benefit. If you look at the table of RS content in various foods (linked in the Resources section), you will quickly conclude that there is no way you can eat all of this every day, especially considering that you would have to consume an awful lot of digestible starch to get the necessary amount of resistant starch. We generally don't have easy access to a lot of the highly fibrous wild tubers and roots that our ancestors chomped on. Thankfully, it's easy and inexpensive to add resistant starch to our daily intake without adding any digestible carbs. There are several ways to do that. Let's start with the simplest and easiest one, almost guaranteed to fit into anyone's schedule or diet.

> *Fair warning: Please do not take the information below to mean that we are advocating the exclusion of real food sources of fiber. We are talking about supplementing, not replacing them. Another: If you have been diagnosed with gut dysbiosis, especially small intestinal bacterial overgrowth (SIBO), taking a resistant starch supplement is not for you.*

Everyone who bakes or makes gravy is familiar with unmodified raw potato starch. Once you use it as a thickener for sauces, soups, and stews and a binder in baking, it turns into your usual starch which (for our purposes) is an enemy. However, if you stir it, raw, into a glass of cold water and add it to your smoothie, cottage cheese, or salad, etc. – you've got resistant starch in its purest form. One tablespoon contains about 8 grams; four tablespoons a day will fulfill your needs.

Let's be smart and careful about incorporating this form into our daily regimen. Start slowly with a half-tablespoon and observe your body's response. The thing is, the process of fermenting the resistant starch may lead to increased gas and bloating. Interpret this effect as the rapid growth of your gut bacteria, which is a very good thing. This side effect, should you observe it, will subside in a few days; add another half-tablespoon then and repeat the process until you get to 3-4 per day. If you feel discomfort, back off and spend a few days with a smaller dose again. If you have no such reaction from the get-go, it most likely indicates that you had a healthy bacteria colony in the first place, so you can start benefitting faster from feeding it.

Aside from taking it alone or mixing it with a smoothie, sour cream etc., there is one more way to utilize its glycemic response mitigating quality. When you are making mashed potatoes the usual way, mix in all of the cold components and let it cool down slightly. Now mix the potato starch into it, about 1 tablespoon per each large potato, and stir well. As long as your mashed potatoes are not hotter than ~140F (the temperature at which potato starch converts into a digestible form), this addition will blunt the blood sugar and insulin spike.

There is one more interesting effect of the resistant starch that we can use to our advantage in a very practical way. Remarkably, RS has a "second meal" effect. That means, not only does it lower your glycemic response (blood sugar and insulin spike) to the meal with RS, but it also does the same for your next meal. I find this fascinating: Your next meal, with no RS in it, will result in a

79

lower spike and your system will return to normal faster. Again, since it almost sounds like some kind of miracle, I'll quote an article from the Journal of Nutritional Disorders & Therapy:

> *"Indigestible carbohydrates have become a common explanation among researchers for the second meal effect. One mechanism by which indigestible carbohydrates is believed to be able to mitigate the glycemic response to a subsequent meal (second meal effect) is through short chain fatty acids (SCFA) created by colonic fermentation."*[*]

In practice, this leads us to the following idea. If you have a high-carb meal later in the day, you can mitigate its effect by taking a couple of tablespoons of potato starch two-three hours earlier. That will blunt the spike and aid in clearing it. Neat, isn't it? Yay for science!

Once again, I want to warn against taking raw potato starch as a substitute for eating fiber-containing plants and other foods. But it is a very good supplement to increase dietary fiber intake and introduce RS in quantities difficult to obtain through food alone. Also, please do not take the second meal effect as permission to eat any quantities of digestible starches or sweets as long as you take RS before that – this trick dulls the spike, it doesn't eliminate it.

---

[*] *The Second Meal Effect and Its Influence on Glycemia*, by Justin A. Fletcher, James W. Perfield II, John P. Thyfault and R. Scott Rector, 2012

Now it's time to introduce another great source of resistant starch that can serve as an actual food. It's filling, adding bulk to your meal and letting you choose your own flavours. Be it teriyaki or soy sauce, eggs or ground meat, stir-fried vegetable or seafood, any spice – you can add it to whatever you like, and it's not going to add any calories. Difficult to believe? Enter **SHIRATAKI NOODLES**. These are made from the konjac yam (also known as devil›s tongue yam or elephant yam). Their main component is glucomannan starch, an indigestible dietary fiber. They are so low in carbs and calories that their oft-used commercial name "zero calories" is actually not a distortion of the truth. They have practically no taste of their own, so they can be made into whatever you want your dish to taste like.

Supermarkets offering Shirataki noodles often have them in different sections so you may have to ask the staff for help locating them. They come in several forms (noodles, pieces, cake) and types – white and black. White is the original form while black (it's actually more like brownish-gray) has some seaweed added to it with additional nutritional elements and a little more flavor.

Using them is very simple. Open the package and dump its content into a colander to drain the liquid. Rinse them well under water – I use hot water since it seems to help decrease the somewhat rubbery texture. Also, while holding them under the water, I cut them with kitchen scissors into shorter strands – that's just how I like eating them.

Please see a gallery at the http://timetraveldiet.com/image-gallery/ for the full color photo illustrating Shirataki noodles.

If you prefer longer noodles, skip this step. Washed well, I dump them on a hot pan without any oil for a few minutes. This step dries them out a bit, further improving the texture. After that, mix them with whatever you'd like. The package that I purchase has a recipe for beef and potato stew on it. Also, the nutrition label displays very satisfactory zeros everywhere:

Nutrition Facts
Valeur Nutritive

Per: 1/14 package (28g)
Par: 1/14 emballage (28g)

Amount Teneur	% Daily Value %valeur quotidienne
Calories / Calories 0	0%
Fat/Lipides 0g	0%
Saturated / Saturés 0g	0%
+Trans / Trans 0g	
Cholesterol / Cholestérol 0mg	0%
Sodium / Sodium 0mg	0%
Carbohydrate / Glucides <1g	0%
Fibre/Fibre 0g	
Sugar/Sucres 0g	
Protein / Protéines 0g	0%

DOESN'T GET MUCH BETTER THAN THIS, DOES IT?

To counter the gelatinous texture, you may want to throw something gritty into the mix. The first thing that comes to mind is something like breadcrumbs... which immediately triggers the thought: wait, what? We spoke of replacements for pasta, for rice, for potato, but we never touched the subject of bread? I would be remiss if I didn't come up with a substitute for that. Remember my suggestion to vary the taste profile of the cassava pancakes with buckwheat and chickpea flour, where I asked you to remember these two and promised to return to them later? The time has come.

BUCKWHEAT AND CHICKPEA BREAD

It took a lot of experimentation. Gluten-free breads can be tricky if you want to reproduce the good texture, density and bind of traditional breads. Knowing buckwheat as a great complex carbohydrate with a healthy dose of protein, fiber, resistant starch and a lot of micronutrients, I really wanted to use it in bread. By the way, did you know that despite having "wheat" in the name, buckwheat is not a cereal or grain at all, but rather a seed, and a relative of rhubarb? It's such a staple in Eastern Europe and so undeservedly under-represented in North American cuisine that I have added a link for it in the Resources section to encourage your interest.

Most of the recipes I could find suggested adding more traditional flours to the buckwheat. I, however, wanted to avoid "all-purpose" and similar flours. Iteration after iteration was taking me gradually closer and closer to the target, until one day my wife said "This is it!"

Please see a gallery at the http://timetraveldiet.com/image-gallery/ for the full color photo illustrating buckwheat bread, 3rd image.

Let's once again cite two variations of the recipe. First is the basic:

- 0.7 litre room temp water (*or whey – remember this remark, we will get back to it*)
- 4.5 Tbsp olive oil
- 1.5 Tbsp vinegar
- 3 eggs
- 2.5 tsp brown sugar

- 2.5 tsp coarse salt
- 2.5 cup buckwheat flour
- 2.5 cup chickpea flour
- 1 Tbsp xanthan gum
- 2 tsp yeast

Set the bread-maker on its Gluten-free setting. My particular model finishes this cycle in 1 hour and 17 minutes.

Please see a gallery at the http://timetraveldiet.com/image-gallery/ for the full color photo illustrating all the ingredients in the bread maker buckwheat bread, 1st image.

After about 10 minutes of mixing, open the lid and look at the surface. To see how it should look at this point:

Please see a gallery at the http://timetraveldiet.com/image-gallery/ for the full color photo illustrating buckwheat bread, 2nd image.

Quite possibly, due to differences in how bread makers mix the dough, it looks differently; there is more dry stuff on the surface. If so, grab a rubber spatula and help the liquid underneath to mix with the upper layer by turning over the portions and scrubbing the sides clean. After the cycle is finished, open the lid and touch the upper crust. It should be just above the rim of the pan, and while the crust itself feels right, you should feel obvious softness underneath. Now put the machine on Bake for 45-50 more minutes. At that point your bread will be ready. Going by internal temperature, your bread is ready at 195-200 degrees F. Depending on the particular model, you may have to experiment a bit to achieve the same result since the Gluten-free mode and the way the machine mixes ingredients varies from brand to brand.

Now let's get fancy and add some interesting ingredients:

1 Add 1-2 Tbsp flax seed
2 ¼ tsp dried oregano
3 ¾ tsp dried basil
4 Add cut black olives, about 1/3 cup
5 Add 2-3 cloves of fresh minced garlic
6 Add 2 Tbsp raw sunflower seeds
7 Add 1 Tbsp of Chia seeds
8 Add 2-3 Tbsp of poppy seeds

I listed here all of the additional ingredients I've tried. You can pick any you like. The bread will be tasty in any case, rich with protein, fiber and other healthy goodness. I love it toasted to a crunchy consistency. The crumbs that you shake out of your toaster are just perfect for those shirataki noodles or sprinkled on top of fried eggs. This 1 ½ pounds loaf will keep on the counter for up to one week (if it survives that long in your home).

Ever since we finalized the recipe, we haven't bought a single loaf of bread from the store. I hope this healthy bread, with its slightly gritty texture and nutty taste becomes a favorite in your family as well. Now, since we have such interesting mix, it would be thoughtless on our part not to make some other goodies with it. Let me add another recipe here, with this comment: There are variety of other flours you can use instead of chickpea, each introducing its own taste and consistency together with buckwheat. Variations we tried include amaranth, tapioca, sorghum and brown rice flours.

OK, enough with the intrigue: **PANCAKES**!

- 1 cup buckwheat flour
- 1 cup chickpea flour (or any of the substitutes listed above)
- 1 Tbsp brown sugar
- 1 Tbsp baking powder
- 1 tsp salt
- 1 tsp cinnamon
- 2 cups buttermilk
- 4 tablespoons (85 grams) unsalted butter, melted
- 3 eggs

Melt the butter in a bowl and stir in the buttermilk and eggs. Mix the dry ingredients in another bowl. Now add the wet ingredients to the dry. Mix them together but without much zeal; it's fine to have lumps, just make sure that there are no dry pieces left. You need the consistency of sour cream; add some buttermilk or either of the flours to thicken or thin out the batter. Add just a tad of oil to the skillet heated to medium and pour the mix in. Cook until the lower side becomes dark-brown (about 3-4 min); flip and cook the other side. I won't recommend syrup on those as it would be against the idea of this whole section, but sour cream or butter is perfect on them... and come to think of it, once we hit our targets with weight and/or diabetes reversal, reasonable portions of syrups or honey could take their place in our diet once again.

Even if you've never tried **BUCKWHEAT CREPES**, you have likely heard of them. With various fillings, from savoury to sweet, they are served in all types of restaurants. Having mastered the recipes in this section, you already have everything you need to make them yourself. There are many recipes on the Internet but we will share just one here, to have everything in one place for you.

- 1 1/4 cups buckwheat flour
- 3 large eggs
- 1/4 cup vegetable oil
- 3/4 cup milk
- 1 cup (or more, depending on the batter consistency) water
- 1/4 tsp salt

Pour the flour in the bowl and whisk in eggs, oil, milk, water, and salt.

Heat a large non-stick skillet over medium-high heat, brushing it with oil. Add 1/4 cup of the batter to skillet and tilt to coat bottom. Cook crepe until golden on the bottom, lifting it to prevent burning, about 30 to 45 seconds. Using a spatula, turn the crepe over; cook for 30 seconds. Transfer to a large dish. Repeat with the remaining batter, stacking crepes on a dish. They can be made a day in advance and kept in the fridge until ready to be filled, heated up and served.

I would like to give you a nudge toward taking a creative approach to any of your favorite foods. With the advent of a wide-spread movement to a healthier lifestyle, few, if any, food choices remained unexamined in attempt to find better equivalents. Most of the recipes are flexible and allow for endless variants in both ingredients and techniques, so feel free to experiment. If you find an undiscovered variation and create your own gem, join the generous sharing community and let everyone benefit! I hope to see your discoveries at http://timetraveldiet.com/

By way of example, let's suppose one of the dishes you enjoy is waffles. I've never made those with any kind of regularity so I never tried to create a buckwheat version myself. If you love them, you can try to construct your own recipe or search for one on the internet. Knowing what a staple it is for many (and remembering what might hide in the store-bought kind), I did search the internet, and found many. Even if you don't come up with a purely wheat-free version, replacing some of it with buckwheat, tapioca etc. will introduce healthier ingredients and new interesting tastes.

Keeping with the spirit of this book, let's again think of something other than syrup or jam for these waffles. Sour cream with blueberries, cream cheese with raspberries? Any other sugarless topping with any berry or fruit? Some butter and cold-smoked salmon? Cross out the sugar from the recipe and add some finely chopped dates, dried apricot or raisins instead.

If your heart is set on cookies, muffins or cakes, you won't be left hanging with no healthy variations for any of those.

As we speak of introducing different ingredients, here is a short guide to some easily found flours. Let this be a starting point for your experiments. Usually flours of this kind are best used in combination rather than single flour per dish. Don't forget to add some xanthan gum to bind the ingredients together. Since these flours are gluten-free, it's necessary in order to prevent crumbling.

Start with small batches to discover the combination you like the most, be it two or four flours in one dish.

High-Protein Flours: Amaranth, Buckwheat, Chickpea, Millet, Oat, Quinoa, Sorghum, Teff.

High-Fiber Flours: Amaranth, Buckwheat, Chickpea, Corn, Coconut, Oat, Quinoa, Spelt, Teff.

Sure enough, you won't face a lack of resources when searching the internet for ideas and recipes.

This would have been a logical place to speak about desserts. We will have to postpone that, however, and there is a good reason for that delay. The next part will familiarize you with a class of foods that will play an important role in some of the sweet dishes.

At this point in our journey, let's pause and have a look at our daily diet:

- We have successfully replaced commercial drinks full of sugar and empty calories with tasty and healthy versions, breaking the dependency on a sugar in the process.
- We found healthier substitutes for many staples in our food; potato, pasta, rice and bread remain in our diet but in a much healthier form.

- We found better versions for pancakes and crepes. Together with the previous point, we have avoided forbidding desirable foods – limitations that make any diet too difficult to sustain.
- We introduced a whole new class of food into our daily regimen – resistant starches that play an enormous role in improving our overall well-being and blood sugar control.
- We formulated a cooling trick to make even traditional starchy products better; we also learned to take resistant starch before carbohydrate-rich meals to mitigate the harmful effects. Together, these take away the pressure of potentially awkward social situations, so that we aren't "that guy" that avoids eating at parties and who keeps referring to his diet.

All these achievements are highly exciting. We are barely over a third of the way through our endeavor, and our blood sugar, weight and overall health are already benefitting noticeably. Part of this benefit should reflect on the bathroom scale, part in blood sugar readings if you are a diabetic. And another, hidden part of the iceberg, is in the preparation of our body for the next steps that will take us much further on this thrilling and highly rewarding path. Just as importantly, we haven't severely limited our food choices making ourselves and our close ones miserable. Instead, we introduced many new tastes and if anything, made our diet more exciting.

Wrapping up this part and transitioning to the next, let's recall one significant concept we encountered earlier. Speaking of resistant starches, we said that they served as a prebiotic – food for our gut bacteria. It's now time to find out more about the role of this bacteria and how to cultivate a healthy colony in our intestines. A few other foods and ingredients mentioned in passing, like cream cheese, whey, butter and some others will take a prominent role in the next section.

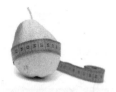

PRACTICAL TAKEAWAY: QUICK SUMMARY

- Replacing potato with cassava, wheat pasta with black beans spaghetti and white rice with parboiled rice sharply decreases amount of starch in our diet.

- Cooling and reheating starchy foods (potato, rice, corn) introduces resistant starches in our food.

- Resistant starch improves numerous functions in our body and serves as a food for our gut bacteria. Second meal effect improves glycemic response of the subsequent meal.

- Resistant starch can be added to our diet with raw potato starch, up to 4 tablespoons a day. Taken a few hours before starch-rich meals, it helps blunt the blood sugar spike.

- Wheat bread can be replaced by buckwheat and chickpea version.

SECOND PRONG:
PLUS BACTERIA

What is your first reaction when you hear the word "bacteria?" The safe bet is that it's germs, sickness, contamination and other unpleasant connotations that spring to mind. We are conditioned to perceive bacteria as something to avoid by means of sanitation and, especially when it comes to food, sterilization. While true in many instances, this view does not distinguish between "bad" bacteria, which brings disease and "good" bacteria, which benefits our body (in some cases even that separation is difficult to make as some bacteria strongly associated with illnesses carry important benefits in other respects). As a result, we sterilize our food and much of our environment, eliminate traditional food preparation processes that promote beneficial gut bacteria, and eat foods inhibiting it. Indiscriminate use of antibiotics doesn't help either.

It's only relatively recently that we started realizing the enormous role good bacteria plays in our gut and overall health. To quote one of the studies on the subject,

> *"Some of the beneficial effect of lactic acid bacteria consumption include: (i) improving intestinal tract health; (ii) enhancing the immune system, synthesizing and enhancing the bioavailability of nutrients; (iii) reducing symptoms of lactose intolerance, decreasing the prevalence of allergy in susceptible individuals; and (iv) reducing risk of certain cancers."*[*]

---

*   J Appl Microbiol. 2006 Jun;100(6):1171-85. *Probiotics and their fermented food products are beneficial for health.* Parvez S1, Malik KA, Ah Kang S, Kim HY.

Another quote I must cite here is from Dr. Mark Hyman:

> "Having a healthy gut should mean more to you than being annoyed by a little bloating or heartburn. It becomes central to your entire health and connected to everything that happens in your body. That's why I almost always start treating my patients' chronic health problems by fixing their guts first.
>
> You can begin to understand the importance of gut health when you consider there are 500 species and three pounds of bacteria in your gut. There are trillions of bacteria in your gut, and they collectively contain at least 100 times as many genes as you do. The bacterial DNA in your gut outnumbers your own DNA by 100 times. You have about 20,000 genes, but there are 2,000,000 (or more) bacterial genes!"[*]

Within the framework of this book and with our main objective in mind, let's state that healthy gut flora aids weight loss, improves metabolism, reduces inflammation and, you guessed it – optimizes the glycemic response.

In case you miss some science-speak as I do now and then, this quote describes what happens when our bacteria feed on resistant starches and produces short-chain fatty acids:

---

[*] *How to Fix Your Gut Bacteria and Lose Weight*, Mark Hyman, MD.

"SCFAs suppress inflammation through GPR43 signalling in immune cells, such as neutrophils, and modulate secretion of the hormone GLP-1 — which improves insulin secretion and has antidiabetic effects — by enteroendocrine L-cells in the distal small intestine and colon." [*]

Here is the good news. By eliminating highly processed foods and foods with added sugars, we removed contents harmful to our gut bacteria. Then we made the next step of adding foods high in fiber and resistant starches – those served as prebiotic food for good bacteria, helping it thrive. One thing that we haven't done yet, which this part of the book is going to describe, is introduce probiotic foods, the source of the bacteria itself.

There are all kinds of capsules and powders that can meet this purpose. I prefer the old-fashioned way, the way our ancestors ate for generations in all corners of the world before the food industry took over and sterilized our food. I am talking about fermented foods, treated and preserved by bacteria, and introducing good bacteria into our gut. Fermented foods have many benefits over supplements, not the smallest of which is that they are amazingly tasty.

Don't be too quick to reach for a yogurt from the store shelf, though. There are more potent and intriguing home-made alternatives, providing a wide variety of probiotics with guaranteed content (which is not always the case with store-bought product).

---

[*] *Functional interactions between the gut microbiota and host metabolism*, Valentina Tremaroli & Fredrik Bäckhed. 13 SEPTEMBER 2012 | VOL 489 | NATURE | 245

The range of products that can be fermented is almost endless. You can find the recipe to ferment anything but a clay brick – and sometimes I think I just didn't search for it thoroughly enough. In this book I will detail those foods that made it into my daily repertoire. They are very beneficial; they don't take a lot of time or great skill to prepare; they offer a cheaper and healthier alternative for healthy bacteria to their store-bought equivalents, and while the taste is always a personal preference, I am yet to find anyone who wouldn't ask for a second helping when trying them at our place. "Oh my, this is the taste from my childhood!" seems to be a frequent reaction to a few of them.

If you're really interested in fermentation, you will discover a wealth of information in the books and sites linked in the Resources section.

Some general words about fermentation and fermented foods. They have been around for centuries, and are very safe. Long before refrigerators, freezers and canning conveyers they served to preserve perishable foods, alter their taste and create new foods with new and different qualities. There are endless variations of the recipes; some differ from country to country, some – from family to family. There are infinite possibilities for experimenting, with various additions and differences in the process, and there is no right or wrong way to do it – it's all about what you prefer. Starting with a basic recipe and then trying different versions is a part of the excitement. Often it's texture and taste that guide you, not the exact weight of the ingredients or precise time of the process. It might feel at first a bit unconventional and even somewhat frustrating to those of us who prefer strict instructions, but it quickly proves stimulating and enjoyable as your creativity gets released. Another unconventional side of fermentation is the somewhat varying results. While the main outcome remains the same and the quality is dependable, differences in the starting ingredients (after all, no two heads of cabbage are exactly the same, right?) and the details of the process like room temperature, can create subtle variations of the finished product's taste – and that, too, is a part of fun. Even definition of the finished product is flexible – you can stop the fermentation on the fifth day, you can let it go for five days more for a different taste, or can start eating it in portions at some point and continue enjoying the changing taste as the process goes on.

As you delve into this ancient technology, you are likely to experience a sense of reproducing some primal ritual, getting in touch with methods and techniques that served our ancestors throughout history. There is something very gratifying about this, recreating ways predating our modern technologies by thousands of years. Just wait until you taste your first fermented food or watch your guests' astonishment when they learn you made this amazing dish yourself; there are few things that create such pride of accomplishment. It's also very exciting to feel yourself being unchained, at least in some aspects, from the standard fare of the food industry. My bet is, store-bought equivalents of some of the foods you ferment at home will taste very bland to you.

Without further ado, let's describe the first of them.

Fermented Sauerkraut

Yes, the humble sauerkraut. If you shrug and think "it's available everywhere and dirt cheap," think again. The majority of the sauerkraut you see on store shelves has nothing to do with fermentation and probiotics. Have a look at the list of ingredients – do you see vinegar or wine there? That's what gives it its sour taste. Even if you see a jar with a label listing nothing but cabbage and salt, if it sits in the usual section of your grocery store at room temperature – rest assured that it has been pasteurized, killing the good bacteria in the process. Real fermented sauerkraut with live bacteria will be found mostly in health stores on refrigerated shelves – and that one won't be anywhere close to cheap.

This is usually the first product recommended to those who are making their first steps in fermenting. We start with it as well, because it's an absolute champion due to its combination of benefits and simplicity of preparation.

Speaking of benefits, where do we begin. Besides the probiotics, sauerkraut is a good source of antioxidants and dietary fiber. A couple of forkfuls a day can give you significant benefits and a great source of nutrients, including vitamin K, vitamin C, calcium, potassium and phosphorus. And the count and variety of bacteria in fermented cabbage is one of the highest among probiotic foods. In fact, it surpasses the over-the-counter probiotic supplements by far. A four- to six-ounce serving, in testing done by Dr. Mercola, showed about 100 times the amount of bacteria compared to a bottle of high potency probiotics. So, you have a tasty food and it delivers significantly more benefits than an expensive capsule – sounds like a no-brainer to me.

As for simplicity, it essentially comes down to shredding a cabbage, adding salt and storing it in a glass jar for a few days. All of the details and steps in the recipe are there to make sure you go through the correct sequence and know what to look for. After you've done it the first time, you'll know there is nothing to it.

There are many variations of sauerkraut in different countries, cultures and even families. It's one of those things that everyone's grandma used to do in her own way. I will describe the way it was done in my native neck of the woods, Ukraine. I like this particular recipe for two reasons. First, it speeds things along; unlike some recipes that may take weeks, if not months to create a well-fermented kraut, this one gets you there anywhere from 3 to 10 days. Second, it produces a crunchy texture, which I find much more pleasant than the soft cabbage shreds that many recipes produce.

As always, let's start with a **BASIC RECIPE** and then list possible variations you can introduce for a variety of tastes.

You'll need a large bowl to mix the shredded cabbage. I use an oval roaster. A sharp knife or a mandoline works well for shredding the cabbage – I prefer a mandoline for speed and protect my hand with a cut-resistant glove. Any shredder will do for the carrots, preferably one with large holes. For the actual fermentation, two gallon-sized mason jars are ideal – you need a wide mouth so you have no troubles packing the cabbage in with your hand. Two average-sized heads of green cabbage and three or four average to large carrots usually fill those two jars about ¾ each, although this will vary depending on their size. You will also need a couple of empty bottles about 0.75 litres that can fit in the mason jars' mouths, to use as a load to keep the sauerkraut submerged.

Before you begin, prepare the brine. Boil some water in an uncovered pot to remove the chlorine (we want the bacteria to thrive, not to die in chlorinated water). Pour one litre of the water into a separate can or jar and mix in 1 1/3 tablespoon of pickling salt (make sure it doesn't have iodine in it) and 1 tablespoon of sugar. (You won't find this ingredient in most recipes, but that's exactly how it has been prepared in some Eastern Europe countries for ages – sugar puts the fermentation process into overdrive and speeds up the process, providing additional food for the bacteria. It doesn't make the finished product sweet though.) Let the water cool down to room temperature.

Cut the cabbage into quarters and remove the core. Remove the outer leaves but do not discard them yet. Now slice the cabbage with your mandoline or a sharp knife to about 1/8" thick strips. Using a large-holed shredder, shred the carrots and mix them in the cabbage. While mixing, try to break cabbage strips – you don't need to turn them into mash or tear them apart, just break them wherever your fingers grab during mixing. This is a bit different from the vigorous pounding that most recipes recommend; this, and introducing a little sugar in the brine allows us to preserve the crunchiness in the finished product while speeding up fermentation.

Now pack your vegetable mix into the mason jar, putting it inside in small portions and packing it tightly. Use your fist or a wooden tool to press it down as much as possible. You want to leave no air pockets. As you do this, the mix takes much less volume than seemed possible; depending on the size of the cabbage heads and thickness of the cut, the whole amount may even squeeze into a single gallon jar. More often, however, about half of it fits in the jar until it's filled up to 2-3 inches under the rim. Pack the rest in the second jar. Now pour your brine in, distributing it between the jars equally. Try to press the mix again so that the brine rises above it, submerging the vegetables and leaving no contact with the air. If not, add some boiled and cooled down water; it shouldn't take more than a cup. Now take those outer leaves you put aside earlier and place them in the jar, creating a layer on top of the mix and separating it from the air. Fill the bottle with water, put it on top of the leaves and press down so that brine rises above the leaves. Now you have a water lock that prevents mold formation.

Put your jars in a tray to catch the overspill that rising brine may create. I use that same oval roaster in which I mix the vegetables. Put the jars away from the sunlight at room temperature (around 70 degrees F is ideal) and let the fermentation do its magic. Once a day, poke the kraut to the bottom using a wooden skewer and inserting it at the side of the leaves that cover the mix. As you do it, you will see bubbles rising toward the surface;

you want to let them escape – that's the purpose of this procedure called burping. On the second day this bubble stream looks quite intense; there is something satisfying about observing this visible sign of the process you initiated, just like your ancestors did centuries ago. About three days in, the intensity of the bubbles will diminish significantly.

Now the fun part starts. Three-four days later you want to start tasting your kraut. There is no exact time when the fermentation is over or the taste is objectively right – you are going to be the judge of it. You are aiming for a tangy tart taste to replace the taste of fresh cabbage; just how tangy it should be depends on your personal preference. The flavor and texture that you deem right is right. When you decide that you have achieved the right taste, cover your jar with a lid and put it in the fridge. For me, this moment usually comes anywhere from 5 to 10 days into the process; a tad longer when the temperature in the house is lower.

When you do it the first time, give it a chance to demonstrate the range of tastes available, by letting the process continue in one portion beyond what you deemed as a finished product. This way you may discover an even more interesting taste for next time. The maturing taste can be quite surprising in fermented products; this process continues even in the refrigerator albeit much more slowly.

It can spend a few months in the fridge; beyond that, the kraut may start losing crunchiness. I personally have never achieved that stage; it's gone long before that, and we start preparing the next portion as our stock dwindles down to about a week's worth of supply. If you left some to sit in the fridge for too long, use common sense to judge whether it is spoiled – a bad smell and taste will unmistakably alert you.

Kraut can be served as a side dish or as a tasty and healthy addition to any meal (well, maybe not to a dessert, although there are some recipes using it even in those!) A forkful or two at each meal became a staple in our household. If you want to use it in dishes that call for heating it up, keep in mind that the bacteria will die above 110 degrees F; you may like the taste, but to obtain the probiotic benefits you need to consume it raw. As you take another portion out, push the remaining kraut down to keep it submerged under the brine and diminish contact with the air. And speaking of brine – try it on its own as a tart drink, quite refreshing in the morning or for helping to settle down any stomach uneasiness. There is a suggestion that it's also helpful for hangovers – hopefully you don't have to check it yourself.

Now that we mastered the basic recipe, let's list a few alterations that introduce a **VARIETY OF TASTES**. There are numerous additions possible that make profound differences in flavor. I recommend trying them on a smaller portion – just set aside some basic mix, enough to fill a quart or a half-quarter jar to test your additional ingredient's influence. When you find your favorite combination, you can then make an entire batch with it, or break it down by a few portions and make fewer versions.

These ingredients are introduced during the mixing stage. *Dill* is a frequent addition to kraut. *Caraway seeds* can also be added– crush 1-2 teaspoons of them per head with a rolling pin and add to the vegetables. Adding some grated *beet* will make your kraut dark red and serve as an interesting addition to a salad. Adding some *garlic* will add an interesting zing to your kraut – just 2-3 cloves per head will have big impact. One of my favorite variations is grated *ginger*, adding a nice, spicy bite. *Bay leaves* or *black pepper* are worthy variations, either by themselves or in combination with others. Adding a few slices of an *apple* introduces some sweetness, contrasting with the sour; it can also lead to a slightly alcohol-like tint, making an interesting twist in the taste. As you read this, you probably think "is there anything I can't try to add to this product?" – and you are correct, there is no limit to what you can come up with. Oregano, bell pepper, sun-dried tomato, coriander, turmeric... let your creative juices flow!

The ways to incorporate kraut into your meals are just as endless, and some of them are quite unexpected. Look in the Resources section for the book with an unsurpassed variety of recipes and uses for this seemingly humble food.

Kombucha

With all of the latest health trends, in all likeliness you have seen and tried the original or flavored kombucha. If so, you are already familiar with this delightfully refreshing, slightly carbonated drink. If not, hold on to your seat, as you are going to be amazed by the taste, the simplicity of making it and by the negligible cost (nothing even close to what you get charged when you purchase the commercial version). We mentioned kombucha earlier when spoke of replacements for carbonated pop drinks; now is the time to get familiar with it.

Kombucha is loaded with probiotics fermented tea, known in many cultures as "tea mushroom" and dating back centuries; the exact origins of the drink are unidentified, which is fitting for something known for a very long time.

There are two ways to brew kombucha at home – in a single batch or continuous brew, which I prefer. The basic way is a single batch method, so let's describe it first. You will need a one-gallon mason jar; 8 bags of black tea (you can use 4 bags of black and 4 of green; just make sure it has no other flavored ingredients or additives, you need pure tea), 1 cup of white sugar, 1 gallon of water, clean fabric (any old towel will do) and 1 SCOBY. A SCOBY is a symbiotic colony of bacteria and yeast, an odd-looking fermenting agent, also known as Mother. You can grow your own SCOBY, although it's easy to find it as those who make their own kombucha pretty soon have a lot of them and give them away or sell them for a few bucks. Look in your local resource for exchange or sale of used goods, and you are likely to find several private and commercial ads. SCOBY will usually be given with some starter kombucha, about 1 cup. See Resources for everything you need to know about SCOBY.

Make sure you do use black tea. You can go for pure black or combination of green and black teas, but green tends to produce weak taste if used alone.

Avoid prolonged contact between kombucha and metal both during and after brewing. This can affect the flavor of your kombucha and weaken the SCOBY over time. Avoid sterilizing the jar and utensils with anti-bacterial soap; use vinegar instead. The same goes for your hands as you handle the SCOBY; those soaps eliminate bacteria indiscriminately, and a "nuke-'em-all" option is not what we need when we are trying to cultivate friendly bacteria.

1 Bring the water to a boil. Stir in the sugar to dissolve, and add the tea. Allow it to steep until the water has cooled to room temperature

2 Once the tea is cool, remove the tea and stir in the starter kombucha. If you don't have any, add ¼ cup of white vinegar. You need the liquid to be acidic to prevent unfriendly bacteria from taking up residence in the first few days of fermentation.

3 Pour the mixture into a 1-gallon glass jar and gently slide the SCOBY into the jar with clean

hands. Cover the mouth of the jar with a clean cloth and secure it with a rubber band. A coffee filter or a paper towel will work as well; cheesecloth might not be sufficient to protect from fruit flies. Most often your SCOBY will float to the top, although it's not unusual for it to stay near the bottom or along the sides of the jar.

4 Keep the jar at room temperature, out of direct sunlight. Ferment for 7 to 10 days, checking the kombucha and the SCOBY periodically. Within a few days you will see a new SCOBY forming on the surface, attached to an original one or separate. If you see brown strings beneath the SCOBY, some sediment at the jar's bottom, and bubbles throughout the liquid, this is all normal and signifies healthy fermentation.

5 After 7 days, begin tasting the kombucha daily by pouring a little out of the jar and into a cup. Don't hesitate to push aside the SCOBY with plastic spoon, it won't mind. When it reaches a balance of sweetness and tartness that is pleasant to you, the kombucha is ready to drink or bottle for the secondary fermentation. Usually this happens between 7 and 14 days – before that it's too sweet, after that it's too vinegary.

6 For secondary fermentation, pour the kombucha into a swing-top bottle (it's the most convenient option but a jar with tight lid will

do as well). Leave a cup of kombucha in the jar as a starter for the next batch. Add a fruit, berry or whatever else you select to flavor your kombucha with, and let it stay at room temperature for 2-3 more days. It becomes carbonated at this stage so be careful not to overdo it, lest your bottle explodes. Move it to the fridge when done. Now, your options for the flavor are nearly endless. Ginger, mango, blueberry, orange zest (one of my favorites), blackberry (the best in my opinion), rose petals, raspberry, strawberry... you get the idea. Any combination of those works as well. Just remember to always add the flavor in the bottle after pouring the kombucha out of the fermenting jar, not to the original liquid itself. You don't need much; a few berries, a tablespoon of thinly cut orange zest or a teaspoon of grated ginger per bottle is enough. Squeeze the berries so they infuse maximum flavor.

7   Now, if you are using a batch method, at this time you already have another mason jar ready with base tea brewed and cooled. Slide the SCOBY with starter in the new jar and repeat the whole process.

Before starting the process for the first time, think it through step by step to make sure you have everything ready, lest you find yourself with SCOBY in your hands and nothing to place it into.

Please see a gallery at the http://timetraveldiet.com/image-gallery/ for the full color photo illustrating kombucha, SCOBY floating on top.

My preferred way to make kombucha is to brew continuously instead of making it batch by batch. This way I have a constant supply of kombucha. I use a larger 2 ½ gallon jar. When the taste reaches the desired tartness, I pour four 500 ml bottles using a jar spigot or, if it's clogged by the yeast, a plastic ladle. By that time I have 2 liters of a new base tea prepared and cooled off, with 4 tea bags and 1/3 cup of sugar. I replace the liquid in the main jar and repeat the whole process for a few days. The exact time, as is usual with fermentation, is a matter of ambient temperature and your personal taste. By the time I pour another portion for the secondary fermentation, the previous batch is already flavored and carbonated, so from this moment on you have an uninterrupted supply.

Please see a gallery at the http://timetraveldiet.com/image-gallery/ for the full color photo illustrating kombucha, sideview of multiple SCOBYs.

It started with one. As you can see on that image, there are a few too many – time to take some of them out and give them away.

The jar sits on top of the freezer which is a warm surface in a generally dark laundry room. If the temperature in the room where you intend to brew your kombucha is low, you may want to put a warming mat under the jar. At one point I even put a string of Christmas lights around it and wrapped the whole contraption in foil.

Please see a gallery at the http://timetraveldiet.com/image-gal-lery/ for the full color photo illustrating what I call the most festive kombucha in the world.

Not only do I like the taste, I also find it a very energizing drink. We often drink it before a long walk or a house chore requiring long sustained effort, and it seems to keep us going for a long time without getting tired.

Kefir

This is one exciting food, in more ways than one. Not only is it unique in its benefits and taste, it also serves as a parent, in a manner of speaking, to so many other foods, each being exceptional in its own right. A staple drink in many Eastern Europe countries, it remains relatively unknown in Western cultures, compared to its sibling, yogurt. Meanwhile, its probiotic count is higher and the range of bacteria is wider; the bacteria in kefir actually colonizes the digestive tract, delivering far broader and longer lasting benefits than the transient bacteria found in yogurt. Add the incredible ease of making it at home at the cost of milk, and you have a real winner.

Kefir is a drink, unlike spoonable yogurt. Its taste is more on the sour side; it also has slight fizziness to it which gave it the nickname "champagne of milk." It's amazingly refreshing; people who have never tried it before usually grow quickly accustomed to it and mention an excited anticipation of having a cup in the morning or before sleep – or both. It's also very versatile as it accommodates almost any added flavor, be it fruit or berry, although most prefer drinking it straight. Its versatility also manifests itself in an extensive variety of delicious products you can make once you have kefir. Just wait until you make your first batch of cultured butter... but I am getting ahead of myself.

The ease of making it is difficult to overstate. In fact, if you can pour liquid from one cup to another, you are qualified to make kefir. That's the extent of skills it takes. Judge for yourself.

You need a fermenting agent called milk kefir grains. Just as kombucha mother, they can be purchased over the Internet or obtained from someone in your local community – grains multiply with time, albeit a bit more slowly than kombucha SCOBY, so folks making kefir start giving them away or selling them for a few bucks when they have more than they need. All you need is a table-spoon of the grains.

Other than that, a 1-litre wide-mouth glass jar, plastic colander and a non-reactive bowl large enough to place a colander in so it sits suspended on the rim is almost all you need; things like a coffee filter or a piece of clean cloth to cover the jar and a rubber band to secure it are pretty much a given with the fermentation pro-cesses. Oh, and milk of course – get whole milk, avoiding skimmed, ultra-pasteurized or ultra-high temperature (UP or UHT) versions. Don't worry about the fat in whole milk; see Resources for studies showing it's safe and beneficial.

Pour the milk in a jar and drop the kefir grains in. They'll float to the top, slightly peeking through the sur-face. Cover the jar with your cloth or coffee filter, secure it with a rubber band and place it away from the sunlight at room temperature. Depending on your taste prefer-ence, the amount of grain and the ambient temperature, fermentation will be over in 12-24 hours. Now place your colander over the bowl and pour the jar's contents in.

Shake the colander a bit so that the kefir strains into the bowl and grains remain in the colander.

Drop the grains back in the jar and pour fresh milk to ferment the next batch. If you don't need it right away, just put the jar in the fridge and take it out when you want to restart fermentation; I put it on such a pause for up to five days and the grains resume their activity without missing a beat. Do not rinse them under water before transferring them to fresh milk; I don't know where this sometimes disseminated advice originated from but it's not a very good idea.

Back to your freshly fermented kefir. You can stir it and put it in the fridge, to drink it when it is cooled to your preference. There is, however, one more step I prefer, which most of the recipes omit. If you pour your kefir in another jar and leave it covered at room temperature for another 4 to 12 hours before placing it in the fridge, it will mature and become fizzy, with a stronger, yet subtle, pleasant bite. That's the step that does justice to that "champagne of milk" moniker. Don't overdo it; you don't want it to separate to a degree where solid and liquid factions become visible. If there is slight separation, just stir it to combine.

After taking the kefir out of the fridge, you will see that it became a bit denser. Stir it thoroughly, let it warm up just a little bit and stir again before drinking. This stirring returns it to its smooth, silky consistency.

That's all there is to making kefir. As you can see, it really is as simple as I promised. In a few weeks you will see that your grains have multiplied and noticeably increased in volume. You have a few options at this point.

You can simply let them ferment your kefir faster; many find that inconvenient though as it breaks their established rhythm of making and drinking the finished product. You can start making more kefir if you need it – that can be handy if you want more of the other products that you can make from it. Or, you can share them with others. Then, you can put them in a separate jar, pour some fresh milk on top and put them in the fridge for two-three weeks. Beyond that, they can be preserved by freezing.

To freeze kefir grains:

- Rinse them well in unchlorinated water;
- Spread them out on a clean towel and cover with another one;
- Place them in the area where they won't be disturbed or contaminated and let them dry well for a day;
- Place them in a zip lock bag and put in the freezer for up to 12 months. Covering them in dry milk powder prevents freezer burn and increases the chances of successful storing;
- To start using them again, defrost them in the fridge and place them in fresh milk. The first few batches may have a slightly "off" taste.

Before we continue, I want to say a few words about those grains. It's a very curious thing in many aspects. They look like a cauliflower floret; to see them, covered in freshly-made kefir:

Please see a gallery at the http://timetraveldiet.com/image-gallery/ for the full color photo illustrating kefir grains.

They are as close to immortality as it gets; unless you kill them by treating them with an anti-bacterial substance, high temperature or prolonged contact with metal, they are practically eternal. In Caucasian countries from which kefir originates, the grains are known to be transferred from generation to generation, living and thriving for an indefinite time. Commercial starter culture, which you can purchase and use to make kefir, has no such viability (it won't be good for more than a few cycles before it stops fermenting) and carries about 1/3 of the number of bacteria strains.

Finally, there is quite a story about how the grains made it out of the Caucasus Mountains into the world. According to the story, the grains were guarded jealously and passed from generation to generation as a part of the family's wealth. Upon learning of the health benefits of kefir at the beginning of the 20th century, members of the All Russian Physician's Society decided to get the famous kefir grains and make the drink available to their patients. Together with Moscow Dairy owner Nikolaj Balandov, they came up with a clandestine plan. A beautiful young woman named Irina Sakharova was sent to the Caucasian Prince, Bek-Mirza Bachorov, to charm him and persuade him to give her the coveted grains. The plan backfired – she was abducted in the local tradition of "stealing a bride" and faced a forced marriage with the prince. A rescue mission saved Irina from the marriage. Facing prosecution, Bek-Mirza obeyed the order to give

Irina what she wanted. Thus, in 1909, kefir grains came to Russia and by the 1930s, kefir was being produced on a large commercial scale in the Soviet Union and became a staple of the Russian diet.

While many prefer drinking kefir straight, it can serve as a base for a smoothie in endless variations, with fruits and berries. Before we speak of that, however, I'd like you to pause and think of this pairing that seems so natural – "seems" being the operative word here. Remember all of the shelves with yogurt, the many brands and varieties? You'll find every conceivable combination in there, fruit or berry or both on the bottom, or on the top, or mixed in, while plain yogurt will represent probably a fraction. But this is a fermented food – and the point of fermentation is bacteria feeding on sugar and converting it, moving the taste toward the tart side of the scale. So, why do we rush to re-introduce sugar into fermented foods? Why do we have versions where the supposed health benefit of low fat masquerades the very real harm of added sugar? The answer is simple, and we dealt with it in a previous section: it's our continental-wide, nation-encompassing sweet tooth, and a misguided belief in the low fat mantra. We identify tasty with sweet, and the sour taste of fermented foods takes us by surprise. Give it a chance to grow on you – but some of us don't. We rush back to the familiar. I've seen this among many guests at our place who tried kefir for the first time. For many the first reaction is "is this supposed to be this sour?" That's followed by "hmmm, I want to try it again" and then by "wow, it grows on me, I like the aftertaste and refreshing feel" – all within five minutes. Some, however, just don't want to deviate from this ingrained notion of sweet being equal to tasty, and want to add familiar components. There is nothing wrong with the occasional use of sweetened combinations, as long as it's actual fruit and berries and not plain sugar, syrup, sweeteners or jams. I just suggest you give the original version a chance and try to grow accustomed to it, and only then add some variety now and then. After banning overly sugary foods from your menu as we've done in the previous section, it shouldn't be difficult or unpleasant for you; chances are, you'll enjoy it very much. To quote Mary Karlin who put it perfectly in her book Mastering Fermentation – Recipes for Making and Cooking with Fermented Foods:

> *"When you ferment a food or beverage for the first time, you may experience unfamiliar aromas, flavors, and textures that develop during the food's transformation... You may be new to that food, without a frame of reference as to how it is "supposed to" smell or taste. Or, it is likely you are unfamiliar with the changes that occur with fermentation. There's a first time for every food or drink we eat. Think of the first time you smelled sourdough bread, or fish sauce, or a "stinky" perfectly ripe cheese. Had you not experienced them previously, you might have thought they were not safe (or desirable) to eat. But, with a tiny taste, they registered as delicious. The tartness of milk kefir, the yeasty aroma of water kefir, or the vinegary sourness of kombucha may be new to your palate. Some you'll love at first sip; others may take a while longer to enjoy. It's all good.*

Knowing that these ferments are beneficial for us often makes it easier to venture into unfamiliar territory more courageously."

Back to our smoothies, they are very simple to make. Drop any combination of fruit and berries in your blender, for instance, banana and blackberry:

Please see a gallery at the http://timetraveldiet.com/image-gallery/ for the full color photo illustrating kefir-based smoothie preparation, 1st image.

Pour kefir on top and pulverize the concoction to the consistency you like (alternatively, use the blender to blend the banana and kefir and then drop the berries in to preserve them whole).

Please see a gallery at the http://timetraveldiet.com/image-gallery/ for the full color photo illustrating kefir-based smoothie preparation, 2nd image.

Gorgeous smoothie with surprisingly refreshing taste:

Please see a gallery at the http://timetraveldiet.com/image-gallery/ for the full color photo illustrating kefir-based smoothie.

Try to add some cinnamon for another twist in taste. Needless to say, any combination of fruit and berries, some blended and some just squeezed a bit or preserved whole, work, and are a real hit with your guests. Peach, cantaloupe, orange, watermelon, peanut butter... run wild with it! If you must add some sweetness, try adding some chopped dates or raisins – those two create an interesting contrast with the sourness of kefir and add a nice change in texture.

Kefir also makes a great salad dressing on its own or with the addition of garlic, your favorite herbs or spices. Its tangy bite is suited perfectly to salad dressings. Before adding ingredients, let the kefir stand in the fridge for a while and carefully pour out some of the liquid on top that separates from the thicker part underneath. This way you will have thicker dressing since kefir tends to change consistency when stirred.

Kefir Cheese

As I mentioned before, once you have kefir you have opened the door to a whole new realm of foods. Kefir cheese is one of them. It's especially good for those remnants of kefir that sat in your fridge for a few days while you still had an uninterrupted supply of fresh batches to drink. I generate such a surplus deliberately by making a quart of kefir daily while we usually drink two cups a day. Thus, every three-four days, I collect enough extra kefir to make a portion of cheese. The cheese will keep in the fridge for about a week.

There are two main ways to make kefir cheese (and of course endless variations with little tweaks, by country, culture and family). Both start with making kefir as usual. The grains go back to culture a fresh portion of milk, and we use only the kefir.

HANGING TO STRAIN

Pour the kefir into a double-layered cheesecloth spread out on a colander, and tie the ends so that the cheesecloth forms a bag that you could hang over a pot or bowl, as shown in the photo, out of direct sunlight. You may want to let the kefir sit in the cheesecloth for 30 minutes or so to make it easier to tie the ends in a bag-like form.

That's it. Now just wait. What happens over the next few hours is the separation of the whey and cheese. Whey, the yellowish liquid that collects in the pot below has many uses on its own; we will get to it shortly. The cheese that remains in the bag changes its consistency depending on the time you leave it hanging. The more liquid that comes out, the crumblier the texture. The first stage is achieved after 5 to 10 hours of hanging, which gives you something resembling spreadable cream-cheese. The closest comparison to a commercial product is a soft cheese known under the trademark Boursin.

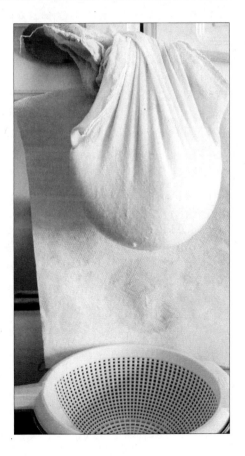

This should start giving you ideas, since there are a few kinds of that cheese on the shelves, and you can approximate them, while having all the benefits of probiotic. One of my favorite savoury combos is sea salt, garlic, black pepper and whatever herbs I happen to have handy – rosemary, basil and oregano make a fantastic mix. Add them all per your taste and mix well; now make the crispy buckwheat bread toast from the previous section and spread this cheese on top. It can also be eaten on its own – I like adding some chopped or crushed nuts into it. Adding cloves works as well.

Sure enough, you can add any fruit and berry. Chopped strawberries and blueberries is one of my favorites. Add some chia or flax seeds for a gritty texture and enjoy one of the healthiest spreads on the planet. Also, try mixing it with cacao powder or adding some cinnamon. Another amazing combination is mashed banana and peanut butter.

Before you try any of the savoury or sweet versions, however, make sure to try the original spread; then add some sea or Himalayan salt for a little kick. Chances are, you will enjoy this spread in its pure form for a while before curiosity takes over and you move on to various versions.

If you leave it hanging overnight, you get a more crumbly texture that lends itself well to adding some salt.

This version is nice to mix with leafy greens (and, optionally, chopped black olives) and sprinkle with balsamic vinegar and/or olive oil for a healthy salad with a probiotic twist. Another intriguing use is to add it to a fruit salad – cut some watermelon, melon, apple, mango (pear, peach and whatever you can think of) and sprinkle crumbs of cheese generously to create an amazing contrast of sour-salty cheese with sweet fruits. Both of these are not unlike how you'd use feta cheese, which this variation of kefir cheese resembles closely.

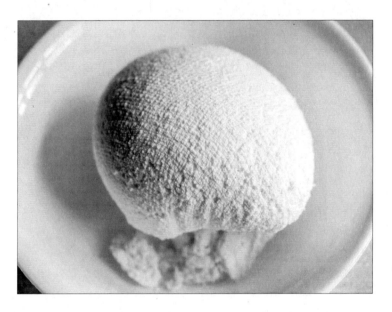

We also like using it as a base for filling white mushrooms. Mix the cheese with some olive oil, salt, a pinch of black pepper, bread crumbs, your favorite herbs and garlic; mash well to create a uniform paste. If you like, you can add shredded shrimp. Measure all the quantities to your taste – there is no right or wrong here. Stuff the white mushroom cups with stems taken out. Sprinkle more bread crumbs on top. Preheat the oven to 375 F and bake the mushrooms for 15 minutes.

A few words about whey. It's an excellent source of protein, used in making protein shakes and bars, and rich in micro-nutrients and vitamins. You can make ricotta cheese with it, but with the quantities we usually have at home it's rarely worth the bother. Still, it's fun and easy, so I added a link describing the procedure in the Resources section. There are many uses for the whey at home. You can add some to your shakes or smoothies, use it as a fermentation starter, a base for refreshing drinks, a meat tenderizer or brine, to acidify the soil for plants that like a lower PH, to make pancakes and even use it as an after-shave, a hair conditioner or a face mask. You will find links with a surprisingly long list of uses for it in the Resources section.

HEATING TREATMENT

This is the second way to make kefir cheese. It gives you a firmer texture and the resulting cheese can better withstand high temperature, which makes it a perfect filling for crepes and for some interesting desserts. Making this version is about as simple as the previous one.

Pour the kefir in the pot and set it on a low heat. Slowly heat it up not letting the temperature go above 160 degrees F. Stir it a couple of times making vertical movements rather than just horizontal, to promote even heating throughout. Watch your kefir to spot coagulation – the moment when the curds separate from the whey. It takes about 20 minutes for me but the exact time depends on the starting kefir temperature and the heat of your stove. If you just took the kefir from the fridge, you can give it an initial nudge by starting at medium heat for a couple of minutes, then turning it down to low heat. Stir while keeping it on medium heat and avoid the temptation to speed up the process by turning the heat up, lest you scorch your kefir.

When you see the coagulation, take the pot off the stove, cover it and let it cool down. When the content reaches room temperature, pour it into the cheesecloth just as you did in the first version and repeat the same hanging procedure, saving and using the whey as before. Cheese will be firmer and somewhat gritty to begin with, and will reach the crumbly state faster, usually in 3-4 hours.

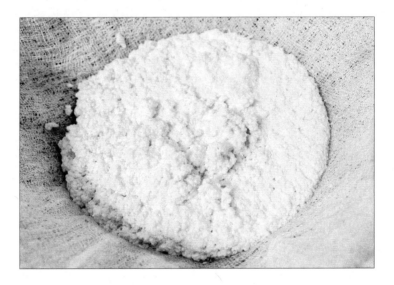

You will notice a somewhat granular texture. From here, you can proceed to try and make it even firmer by placing the bag in the bowl and putting pressure on it overnight – for instance, set a large plastic can of vegetable oil on top of it. Fill the bowl with pressed cheese with a mix of salted water with whey which results in a cheese closely resembling feta.

Please see a gallery at the http://timetraveldiet.com/image-gallery/for the full color photo illustrating home-made feta cheese on lettuce with cranberries.

If you don't want to turn it into feta, you can use it with all the mixes and add-ons we listed for the hanging version, except it's not as suitable as a spread. Also, now is a great time to reach out for that buckwheat crepe recipe from the Second Prong. Make those crepes and use this cheese as a filling, in this case with cranberries added (don't let this image stop you from adding raisins, cinnamon or whatever your fantasy suggests):

Please see a gallery at the http://timetraveldiet.com/image-gallery/ for the full color photo illustrating buckwheat crepes with cream cheese filling, 1st image.

Wrap the crepe like an envelope and heat it up on the pan with a drizzle of oil. You can serve it with a dollop of sour cream.

Please see a gallery at the http://timetraveldiet.com/image-gallery/ for the full color photo illustrating buckwheat crepes with cream cheese filling, 2nd image.

Wait... sour cream? Did you just get up to go to a grocery store for that? Don't.

SOUR CREAM

Your kefir is a powerful fermenting agent that turns milk products into delicious probiotics, comparable to those you buy in the stores. Here comes one of those, and it couldn't be easier to make.

All you need is 18% cream and some kefir. Pour the cream in a glass jar and add finished kefir, 1 Tbsp per 1 cup of cream. Use a whisk to stir your mix vertically, moving it up and down through the volume of the cream to make sure that you distribute the kefir through the entire height of the jar. Place the covered jar in a warm place out of direct sunlight and leave it for 12 hours. Then start checking on the scent and consistency – you want to see a texture close to that of sour cream and it should have a recognizable tangy smell. Sometimes it's finished in 12 hours and sometimes it can take up to 48; my average seems to be about 24. After the desired state is achieved, put it in the fridge where it's going to thicken a bit. Done.

One important thing to know here: If, after a few hours in the fridge it thickens to a desirable consistency but you find the sour taste lacking, simply put it out in the warmth again and give it 12 more hours. It's a pretty bullet-proof process in that you can make corrections until your optimum flavour is achieved.

Now, along with sour cream there is an interesting version of a cream-based, tangy product. Read on.

CRÈME FRAICHE

Crème Fraiche is more delicate and rich in flavor, while slightly less tangy, than sour cream. It's also a bit thicker. I prefer it when used with dessert; you may try both and decide which is more suitable for various uses. Make sure you focus on the complex aftertaste as it changes for a few seconds after making its way through your palate. It's also a mouthful, thanks to a high fat content, so you are likely to eat less of it.

The way you make this one is exactly the same as sour cream. The only difference is that you use 33% whipping cream instead of 18%. That's all.

The time required to reach the desired taste again depends on the temperature, fermenting culture and your taste. The longer you keep it, the sourer it becomes, moving from the cream to the sour cream side of the scale. I kept it for as long as 48 hours once, and loved the bite. The first time you make it, you may want to separate it into several smaller portions and let those mature to different stages, from 12 to 48 hours. Taste, and decide which one suits you more.

For both sour cream and Crème Fraiche you can use buttermilk instead of kefir to culture the initial cream. Where do you get buttermilk? This is where we get to one of the best foods you can make with your kefir.

Cultured Butter

You may have tried it under the name Old Fashioned, European Style, Antique, or some variation thereof. If you are lucky enough to hail from one of those village families that had access to unpasteurized milk, you may also know it under the name "Oh my God, this is how my Grandma's butter tasted!" It has a deeper yellow color than most freshly churned butters and a distinctive, slightly tangy taste.

Keep in mind that industrially-made cultured butter is not guaranteed to be the real thing since some of them are flavored rather than cultured, by simulating the taste with added compounds. As is often the case, making it yourself means you know exactly what's in it. And, as has been the case with all of the foods we discussed on these pages, it's surprisingly simple to make. I make a months-worth stock of the butter at once, and it takes me about 40 minutes of hands-on time, clean-up included.

I list the quantities I use; re-calculate them for your needs. You will need whipping cream with the highest fat content you can find (in Canada it's 33%), kefir, sea salt, a 1-gallon mason jar, a hand mixer (unless you already own a stand mixer), a large bowl, a rubber spatula, a plastic colander and a roll of wax paper.

First, you need to culture the whipping cream. Pour 3 liters of it in the jar and add 9 Tbsp of kefir. 3-4 Tbsp per liter or 1 Tbsp per cup is a good rule of thumb when you calculate your quantities. During the hot season, use 3 Tbsp; if the temperature in your house is on the cool side, make it 4. To make the mixing easier and make sure that culturing agent is distributed throughout, I alternate them when fill the jar: 1 Tbsp of kefir, a half-liter of cream, another Tbsp of kefir etc. Whisk well, agitating the cream vertically. Cover with a coffee filter or a towel and culture for 12-24 hours, using your nose as a guide. A pleasant, slightly tangy scent is what you are aiming for. If you are not ready to start making butter when your cream is cultured, just put it in the fridge. You want both the cream and the mixing bowl cold, so put the bowl in the fridge as well.

Before churning, think through the entire process and make sure that you have everything handy. When you start massaging the butter, your hands will be covered in it and reaching for something you forgot to prepare will be the kind of thing they film for comedies. The best way to handle it all is to have your better half nearby to cheer you on and to help you when you need a couple more hands.

Wash your hands, avoiding anti-bacterial soap. Now pour the cream in the bowl, making sure that you leave at least an inch of headroom – the cream will rise during whipping. Start whipping with your mixer on the highest speed possible without splattering the cream. In a few minutes it will thicken and create firm peaks:

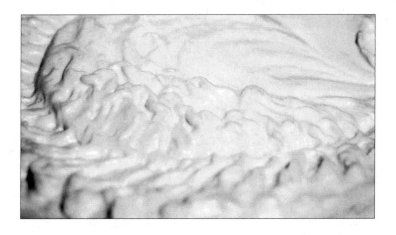

At this point increase the speed to maximum. Watch for the moment when yellow butter balls separate from the white liquid and you hear gentle splashing; at this point decrease the speed to minimum and churn for just a minute more. The whole process takes me under 10 minutes. To see how it looks at this point:

Please see a gallery at the http://timetraveldiet.com/image-gallery/ for the full color photo illustrating separation of butter and buttermilk.

Now, put a colander over a pot and carefully pour the white liquid in, trying to hold the butter with one hand. A colander will catch the butter that escapes. After pouring it all out, sit the bowl on a flat surface and start folding the butter over itself with your hand, squeezing the liquid out and pouring it in that same pot. We will get back to this liquid in a few moments.

When you can't squeeze any more liquid, pour some cold water over the butter and continue pressing and massaging it. Now you are just washing your butter, so when the water becomes milky, pour it in the sink. There is something very satisfying about this process, I have to say. I don't view it as a chore and rather enjoy every minute of it. Continue doing it until the water runs clear and you can't press out any more white liquid. Pour some clear water in once or twice just in case. When there is nothing but butter left in the bowl, massage it vigorously to squeeze out the last remaining clear water, and pour it out.

If you want unsalted butter, sprinkle just a tad of sea salt and mix well. It won't make your butter salted; it will just amplify a flavor a bit. You did prepare some salt on the counter so you can pinch it with your fingers, right? Because if not, there is no way you can use a salt shaker with your hands all covered in butter; that's the moment when you ask your significant other for help. If you want salted butter, increase the salt according to your taste.

This is also the moment when you can add garlic and herbs, should you wish to make this variation. Usually I do that when ¾ of the unsalted butter is wrapped and I have ¼ remaining in the bowl. A mix of salt, garlic and rosemary is a hit in my household. As always, let your imagination run free. Parsley, chives, tarragon, pepper, finely grated lemon zest, basil, thyme, sage, oregano, marjoram... I'll stop now. Just don't forget to mark the wraps with flavored butter.

Your butter is ready for wrapping now. Put a handful of it on a piece of wax paper:

Please see a gallery at the http://timetraveldiet.com/image-gallery/ for the full color photo illustrating cultured butter, before wrapping.

Now wrap it to form a small log:

Please see a gallery at the http://timetraveldiet.com/image-gallery/ for the full color photo illustrating cultured butter, wrapping.

Use a rubber spatula to scrape the remaining butter from the walls of the bowl; there is a surprisingly large amount of it even though it looks like a thin film. With the same spatula get the last pieces of the butter off your fingers. When done, look around to make sure no one is watching and lick them clean.

I keep the butter in the fridge for up to a month. Its taste slowly develops and becomes even richer as it matures. If you need to keep it longer, put it in the freezer for a few months. I have yet to do it; it has no chance of surviving hungry hosts and guests for that long. Spread this butter over a slice of buckwheat bread toasted crisp and you'll understand. I also like to take it out of the fridge in advance so it has a chance to warm up, soften a bit, and reveal its taste to the fullest:

Please see a gallery at the http://timetraveldiet.com/image-gallery/ for the full color photo illustrating cultured butter.

Ever since I started making cultured butter, we haven't purchased a single stick at the store. When you have your first bread-and-butter snack with your own bread and your own butter, take a pause after the first bite and marvel at the thought of unchaining yourself from another industrially made class of foods – cream cheese, soft cheese, sour cream, Crème Fraiche and now butter. Just how good does it feel?

Back to that white liquid. That's buttermilk – pure and traditional, a by-product of making butter, unlike the store-bought version, which is made from skimmed milk. There are a few uses for it. Traditionally, it's used to make pancakes. When you make fried eggs, add a splash of buttermilk to the mix for the luxurious texture and a pleasing twist in the taste. You can chill it and drink it on its own – it's nicely sour and refreshing. Some add black pepper to it. Finally, it can be used as a fermenting agent instead of kefir for any of the foods we discussed earlier, including your next portion of this same butter – it's just as full of probiotic bacteria.

Have you ever suspected you could make that many intriguing foods out of a simple bottle of milk?

Just in case the idea of using dairy fats bothers you, let me offer this quote from The Obesity Code by Dr. Jason Fung:

> *A comprehensive review of all the studies of high-fat dairy finds no association with obesity, with whole milk, sour cream and cheese offering greater benefits than low-fat dairy. Eating fat does not make you fat, but may protect you against it. Eating fat together with other foods tends to decrease glucose and insulin spikes.*

Now that we have kefir, sour cream and cultured butter, let's construct a very gut- and blood sugar-friendly side dish:

MASHED SWEET POTATOES WITH SOUR CREAM AND BUTTER

Wash sweet potatoes (about 2 pounds) but do not peel them. We want to preserve the skin with its influence on the drastic improvement of the glycemic response. Cut them into ½ inch cubes. Cook in boiling water for about 20 minutes until fork-tender. Drain water and mash well, not leaving any lumps. Add 2 Tbsp butter and mash together. Add ½ cup sour cream and mash again. If it's still too thick, add a few Tbsp of buttermilk. When achieve the consistency you like, add salt and pepper to taste; I also like to add some garlic. If you need to heat up the leftovers the next day, try a frying pan instead of microwave – it will add nice crispy crust.

FERMENTED BUCKWHEAT BREAD AND PANCAKES

Let's circle back to our bread and pancakes made with buckwheat flour. In the spirit of the section devoted to fermented foods, we can introduce another variation made with whole buckwheat and put through the fermentation process. I stumbled onto this recipe on the website of a Canadian catering company specializing in whole plant-based food. First, a quote from the website, with insignificant clarifications:

Ingredients
- 3 cups whole buckwheat groats (not the roasted buckwheat also known as kasha)
- ½ -1 tsp salt (quality unrefined sea salt or Himalyan salt)
- Non-chlorinated water

137

- Coconut oil or quality sunflower oil(for greasing pan)
- Sesame seeds or poppy seeds (optional)

Instructions

1 Rinse the buckwheat, cover with two inches of water and soak overnight

2 In the morning drain the buckwheat (water will be mucilaginous/slimy); do not rinse; leave the grains resting in a sieve for up to a minute

3 Combine the buckwheat with ¾ -1 cup of fresh water and salt and blend in food processor or with a hand blender. Blend for at least 1-2 full minutes or until there are no more visible pieces of buckwheat

4 Pour the batter (which should be pancake batter consistency) into a glass or plastic bowl, cover with a clean dish cloth and leave out at room temperature for approximately 24 hours to ferment

5 The next morning your batter is ready for use. If not using immediately, store batter in fridge for up to 4 days

6 Preheat oven to 400 degrees F. Grease glass loaf pan and sprinkle the bottom and sides generously with seeds (or use parchment paper)

7 Pour batter into pan, place in oven and reduce heat to 350 degrees F. Bake for 1 hour

8 Remove from oven and allow bread to cool for at least 1 hour before removing from pan. Once completely cool, slice bread, enjoy toasted

Tips and troubleshooting:

- If in a hurry, soaking for 2 hours can be sufficient and fermenting time can be reduced to 8 hours especially in a warmer environment
- Fermenting can be done directly in the greased baking pans
- If bread does not have air holes once baked the issue may be related to the blending time. If using a food processor, it is important to blend it long enough. If using a high powered blender, it is important not to over blend. Otherwise it may be a matter of oven temperature. Try keeping the temperature at 375 and bake breads on a higher oven rack
- Once sliced, wrap the bread in baking paper (or paper towel to keep moisture off the bread) and then place into a bag. Store in the fridge for 7-10 days or freeze. Once ready to enjoy...toast the bread until edges are golden brown
- For large square slices, bake the bread in an 8×8 inch (or 9×9) glass pan and reduce the baking time slightly. Cut into four squares and then cut each square in half

Variations and alternate uses

(excluding the first option, these variations are all to be applied after step 4 in the instructions)

1 Replace up to one third of the buckwheat in the batter with separately soaked quinoa
2 ***The batter makes great pancakes!*** *We add*

*cinnamon and shredded coconut then scoop
into a hot, oiled, cast iron pan. Allow to cook
thoroughly on one side before flipping. The
batter can also be watered down to make
excellent crepes or wraps*

3   *Add 1-2 cups of seeds. Our favorite is a mix of
sunflower and pumpkins seeds (which have
been soaked for 4-10 hours and rinsed) with
more sesame and poppy seeds*

4   *Add ½ cup sliced olives and ½ cup sundried
tomatoes pieces*

5   *Add ½ tsp. cinnamon and ½ cup each of
shredded apple, raisins and coconut*

6   *Makes a fantastic pizza crust: grease a baking
sheet, sprinkle with sesame seeds, pour batter
on thinly and pre-bake for 10-15 minutes before
adding toppings*

7   *Try using this base to replace the flour, eggs
and milk in your favorite cake recipe
http://consciouscatering.ca/nama-bread*

Now a few comments and photos from me. It probably depends on many variables, but my baking time and temperature are higher; I need to bake it at 400 F and it takes about 90 minutes. I watch for the surface to look like a cracked desert surface and a golden-brown color. If in doubt, try to take the temperature by inserting the kitchen thermometer in the middle of the loaf; a reading of 190 to 200 F indicates that your bread is ready. I also prefer it a bit saltier, but the time to add some more salt is after the fermentation, before pouring the batter in the baking pan; that's also when I add other ingredients when I want to flavor the bread. My favorite variations are:

- Raisins, dried cranberries and crashed walnuts;
- Sunflower and pumpkin seeds;
- Roasted garlic, cut black olives and oregano.

A few images to give you an idea of what to look for:

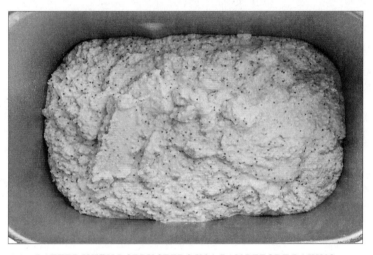

BATTER WITH POPPY SEEDS IN A PAN BEFORE BAKING

After baking; you can see that "cracked desert" look:

Please see a gallery at the http://timetraveldiet.com/image-gallery/ for the full color photo illustrating fermented buckwheat bread, surface.

To see how it looks when cut, with those air holes creating a perfect texture:

Please see a gallery at the http://timetraveldiet.com/image-gallery/ for the full color photo illustrating fermented buckwheat bread, cut.

It doesn't rise much, so it will be flatter than your usual bread loaf.

Pancakes with added cinnamon and shredded coconut come out crispy if you use the same consistency as for the bread, and can be made fluffier if you add water or buttermilk. To see the crispy version:

Please see a gallery at the http://timetraveldiet.com/image-gallery/ for the full color photo illustrating fermented buckwheat pancakes.

They beg for sour cream on top, and if you want a sweet topping, fresh berries can't be beat:

Please see a gallery at the http://timetraveldiet.com/image-gallery/ for the full color photo illustrating fermented buckwheat pancakes with blackberries.

Desserts

Getting rid of harmful sugary foods and adding fermented foods to our diet are two main themes of this book thus far. Hence, it would only be logical to offer some ideas for desserts accomplishing these two goals.

All of them are simple. Some of them are obvious. Most of them amount to a combination of the foods we already mastered. The majority of them include no added sugar, with the rare exception when honey is needed for fermentation. Most of them have distinctive tastes, combining healthy, sweet flavours with the tartness of ferments.

I want to make an important point here. Every time a recipe or a food combination calls for sweetness, I want to use natural sugars with all their benefits – fiber, vitamins and other micronutrients. Thus my first go-to is fresh fruit and berries. Second in line would be their dried versions – dates, raisins, and chopped, dried fruit. Since commercially available dried fruits often have sugar added, I try to make some of my own, by dehydrating or freezing pears, apples and grapes during their natural growing seasons. Only if no such option is available will I add some brown sugar, honey or agave/ maple syrup. That said, keep in mind that sugar plays a role in the structure of ice cream, influencing the formation of ice crystals. Replacing it makes the process somewhat unpredictable, so try to make a small batch first to test the result. It's just fine with me, as I view such experimenting as part of the fun and don't mind a non-traditional texture.

This collection doesn't pretend to exhaust the ideas – it aims to help you generate them.

NO ADDED SUGAR BAKED APPLE

Granny Smith is my preferred apple for this dessert. It presents a more interesting combination of sweet and sour than yellow-red varieties.

Preheat oven to 350 degrees F. If using a counter-top oven, set it on medium heat. Scoop out the core from the top with a peeler or a sharp knife with a thin blade. Make sure not to cut all of the way through – you want to make a narrow well in the apple, so aim to stop where you've removed all the seeds. Drizzle the insides with cinnamon. Optionally, add some nutmeg. Now stuff the well with cheese – elect either the "heated" variety or feta among those we mastered earlier. They withstand the temperature better than a strained variety. Bake for about 15 minutes. The exact time depends on the size of your apple and the tenderness you want to achieve. Both a tender spoonable consistency and a bit firmer texture have their fans, so experiment with it when you bake them for the first time to find out what you prefer.

One interesting variation of this recipe is to replace cheese with one teaspoon of butter. Another idea is to stuff the apple with crushed walnuts and cover with one spoon of cheese, pushing it in like a plug. Have fun with other versions and enjoy your guests' amazement when they discover just how simple, yet delicious, such a healthy dessert can be, while consisting of such common ingredients. Oh, and don't forget to put a dollop of chilled Crème Fraiche on their plate – it presents a fantastic contrast of cold and hot, tangy and sweet. In a way, it reminds one of a more conventional combination of hot pie and ice cream, in a much healthier form of course.

NO ADDED SUGAR BAKED PEAR
While this sounds similar, it's prepared a bit differently. Pick firm pears for this dish; slightly under-ripened ones work the best, as they don't get mushy.

Preheat the oven to 350 F. Cut the pears in half. Cut the bottom of each half, just a little, so it can stand on its own. Scoop out the core with a tablespoon or a peeler. Optionally, put a few drops of a cooking wine in the well – dry sherry works the best. Drizzle the pear with cinnamon. Now fill the well with cheese and sprinkle some crushed walnuts on top. Set it in the oven for 20-25 minutes. A few fresh berries on top will add to both the appearance and taste. Serve with chilled sour cream or Crème Fraiche.

Before we move on to the next recipe, a couple of comments about these two recipes. First, do not peel the apples or pears – as strange as it may seem, there are recipes out there that call for that. Second, it amazes me that the majority of recipes for baked apple and pear call for sugar, honey or syrup; but we know better by now, don't we? The sugar that our fruit contains naturally is more than enough.

FRESH FRUIT AND BERRY SALAD WITH CRÈME FRAICHE

This one is a bit embarrassing. I mean, do you really need a recipe to throw together a few of your favorite fresh fruits and berries and add some Crème Fraiche on the side or on top? Cut the fruit into bite size pieces; if you use strawberries, cut them too. Blueberries, blackberries and raspberries all taste amazing with this topping. You can try some cinnamon, but don't overdo it.

ROASTED PEACHES AND PLUMS WITH CRÈME FRAICHE

A few peaches and plums, halved and pitted, and a few tablespoons of unsalted butter are about all you need as a base for this dessert. Preheat oven to 375 F. Melt the butter in a skillet with an all-metal handle – the kind you can put in the oven. If you like, you can add some thyme at this stage. Add peaches and plums, cut side down, and cook them without stirring for 2 minutes over high heat. Take the skillet off the heat and turn the fruit over; then transfer the skillet in the oven and roast for about 4-5 minutes. Take it out of the oven, transfer the fruit on the plate and pour the sauce remaining in the skillet over the plums and peaches. Serve with Crème Fraiche on the side or on top. I like to have it on the side for a hot dessert, so it remains chilled right up to the moment of being eaten.

ROASTED PUMPKIN WITH CRÈME FRAICHE

Preheat oven to 375 F. Cut the pumpkin into cubes, about 1-2 inches thick, or to wedges if it's on the smallish side. Put them on a cooking tray lined with foil, drizzle with olive oil, crushed walnuts and cinnamon. Cardamom and/or cloves are optional if you like them. Roast about 35-40 minutes, until fork-tender. Serve with Crème Fraiche.

As an interesting twist, add a few Granny Smith apples cut to wedges in the last 10 minutes. They'll be a bit firmer than pumpkin, creating a nice, contrasting texture.

You can also turn it into puree in a blender or food processor or even add garlic and black pepper for a spicy dish – but that wouldn't be a dessert anymore, would it?

DATES WITH CHEESE

Preheat oven to 350 F. Line the cooking tray with foil or wax paper. Open the dates and stuff them with cheese of a firmer variety, then press sides together to close. Bake them for about 10 minutes.

Interesting variation turns this dish into an appetizer. Wrap the stuffed dates in a piece of bacon or prosciutto. Use a wooden toothpick to hold it together. Bake for 15 minutes, turning once midway. Count on 3-5 dates per guest at least, they tend to disappear in a hurry. Just ask my daughter, who originally gave me an idea for this recipe.

NO SUGAR ADDED NO MILK BANANA-CHOCOLATE-STRAWBERRY ICE CREAM

This dessert is based on the interesting properties of a banana: frozen and pureed in a food processor or a blender, it turns into a silky creamy custard-like substance which constitutes a perfect base for an ice cream imitation. From there, you can add any ingredients for any flavor you can think of, so take this chocolate-straw-berry combo as a starting suggestion and create endless variations with your favorite fruits and berries.

Pick ripe bananas for this dish. One large banana will result in about one cup of ice cream. Peel it and cut into chunks small enough to be pulverized in your food processor. I used a blender for this and chunks about ¼ inch worked well. Put the pieces in a freezer bag or any airtight container; freeze overnight. If you are in a hurry, 2-3 hours might be enough.

If after trying a few recipes for this dish you decide you want to make it on a regular basis, you may want to purchase a dedicated frozen treat dessert maker. It's a relatively inexpensive small kitchen appliance which works well and delivers better and more consistent results. Start with what you have, though, and progress from there.

Drop the frozen pieces in your blender and use the pulse setting to crush them. Let them thaw a bit first (10-15 minutes should be enough) – when frozen solid, they may be too difficult for your appliance and possibly even break it. If crumbled pieces stick to the walls, scrape them down and blend further. Repeat the process a few times, not leaving any chunks of banana. You will see the consistency changing from crumbles to mush to creamy texture. When you get this silky cream, blend 10-20 seconds more to whip in some air – that will make it less dense and resembling the familiar texture of aerated ice cream. Add a teaspoon of cocoa powder and chocolate chips and blend to create a uniform color. You can add chocolate chips last and just mix well instead of blending if you want them to remain chunky.

Chop the strawberries into small pieces and stir into the mix. Alternatively, you can add strawberries during blending to get more uniform blend vs. small bits mixed in – it's a matter of a personal preference. Transfer your ice cream to a container; cut one strawberry into larger slices and insert them on top to decorate the dessert; sprinkle a few chocolate chips on top. Return it to the freezer for 10-15 minutes if you want a firmer ice cream, or eat right away if you like a softer consistency.

Let's compare the nutritional data. 100 grams of conventional ice cream is about 21 g of sugar and 207 calories; our banana imitation is 12 g of sugar and 89 calories. 3 g of dietary fiber vs. 1 in ice cream, glycemic load 8 vs. 12. You get the picture.

To throw out a few ideas and jump-start your creativity: Try adding peanut butter to your banana base; almonds, cinnamon, coconut shreds, chopped dates, any berries, mint... alternatively, walk through the ice cream aisle and read the labels for ideas. Leave proudly without buying any of that highly processed stuff full of pois... umm, I mean high fructose corn syrup, and go home to make a healthy, delicious sibling.

Adding some buttermilk or kefir is very much worth checking out. It changes the taste profile toward an intriguing mix of sweet and tart; adding some cinnamon makes it really interesting. You can either add kefir in a liquid form, moving the consistency toward a smoothie, or freeze it in an ice form and keep a soft-serve, ice-cream feel.

You can try any other frozen fruit instead of banana, but expect the outcome to be more of a sorbet rather than ice cream.

(Speaking of sorbets, let me show you what you get when purchase one from the store shelf:

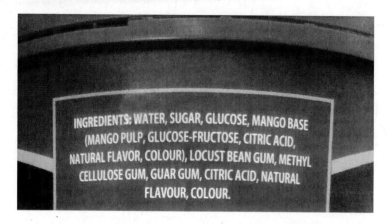

INGREDIENTS: WATER, SUGAR, GLUCOSE, MANGO BASE (MANGO PULP, GLUCOSE-FRUCTOSE, CITRIC ACID, NATURAL FLAVOR, COLOUR), LOCUST BEAN GUM, METHYL CELLULOSE GUM, GUAR GUM, CITRIC ACID, NATURAL FLAVOUR, COLOUR.

Doesn't it astonish you that out of fourteen ingredients only one is actually food? Feel like making it yourself rather than eating sugar, glucose and glucose-fructose, generously sprinkled with natural flavor and coloured for your viewing pleasure? Thought so).

One very worthy addition to any of these, and many other dessert ideas, is toasted, unsweetened, shredded coconut sprinkled on top or even stirred in. To toast it, preheat oven to 325 F, spread coconut flakes on the baking sheet and bake for 5-10 minutes stirring once or twice to ensure an even golden-brown color and a nice crispy texture. Full of healthy fats and fiber, it's a great addition, albeit high on a caloric side.

SOUR CREAM, KEFIR AND CRÈME FRAICHE BASED ICE CREAM

I found these recipes online and used them with no or minimal modifications other than not adding any sugar to those that contain berries. Thus, I'll simply link to them and list modifications where I did make them. Notice that there are variations for an ice cream maker and for manual on these pages.

- http://www.culturesforhealth. com/learn/recipe/cream-recipes/ creme-fraiche-vanilla-ice-cream
- http://www.culturesforhealth. com/learn/recipe/cream-recipes/ strawberry-sour-cream-ice-cream

In kefir ice cream, I have added some dark chocolate chips and toasted pecans:

- http://www.culturesforhealth.com/learn/ recipe/milk-kefir-recipes/kefir-ice-cream

A few more; in these I have used about 1/3 to ½ of the amount of sugar in recipes, and they worked perfectly. I suppose my adjusted sensitivity to sugar played a role, although none of those who tried them at our place ever mentioned a lack of sweetness:

- http://www.culturesforhealth.com/ learn/recipe/milk-kefir-recipes/ chocolate-chip-raspberry-kefir-ice-cream

- http://www.culturesforhealth.com/
  learn/recipe/milk-kefir-recipes/
  apple-cinnamon-kefir-ice-cream

The following recipe I tried both as described and with added toasted shredded coconut, and the crunch and taste variation were very much worth the experiment:

- http://www.culturesforhealth.com/
  learn/recipe/milk-kefir-recipes/
  lemon-blueberry-kefir-ice-cream

In this one I added chocolate chips and a few roasted coffee beans for an amazing crunch:

- http://www.culturesforhealth.com/
  learn/recipe/milk-kefir-recipes/
  coffee-kefir-ice-cream

Chocolate kefir popsicle, amazing in hazelnut version:

- http://www.culturesforhealth.com/
  learn/recipe/milk-kefir-recipes/
  chocolate-kefir-ice-pops

FERMENTED CRANBERRIES

This is one unconventional dish – sweet, sour and slightly alcoholic. Until you try it, anything I say to describe it won't do it justice. My bet is, once you make it you will want to have it in your menu frequently.

You will need a pound of whole cranberries, zest from one large orange, a 2-inch long piece of ginger root, 2 Tbsp of raw unpasteurized honey, 1 Tbsp of whey as a starter (desirable but not necessary), 3-5 whole cloves, 1 cinnamon stick and 1/2 tsp of sea salt. Prepare some unchlorinated water by boiling it in an open pot and letting it cool down to room temperature.

Pour cranberries in a bowl and smash them up a bit with a sturdy potato masher. Alternatively, put them in a zipper or any other bag and smash with whatever is heavy and handy enough. What you want is to achieve is mostly whole berries with their skin popped. Some will remain unpierced but most should be burst. Pour them in 1-liter glass jar. Pour 1 Tbsp of whey on top – it will jump-start the process but if you don't happen to have any, don't worry; honey and water will do the trick.

Remove as much pith from orange zest as you can. Alternatively, zest orange leaving pith behind – that white spongy stuff has a bitter taste that we don't need. Cut the zest in thin strips and tear them with your fingers. Grate the ginger. Mix zest, ginger, salt and cloves and pour the mix in the jar. Break the cinnamon stick in two-three parts and put them in the cranberries. Pour the honey in the jar. Fill the jar with water up to an inch under the rim. Cover with a lid and shake the whole thing vigorously to mix ingredients well. Unscrew the lid and press the mix down to submerge the berries. Cover with a towel and secure with rubber band. Alternatively, put a lid on it without screwing it at all – that's my preferred way. During fermentation the level of the liquid will rise, and you may not always be able to catch it in time to prevent spilling. Put the jar in a dish to collect the spillover. Place it away from direct sunlight.

In a few days you will see bubbles in the liquid. In about a week you may start tasting the berries. They will be much more mellow than cranberries usually are and slightly fizzy. I usually eat some while leaving the rest to ferment further and mature in taste – as with most ferments the taste develops and changes with time. You can stop the taste change at any time by putting the jar in the fridge.

THIRD PRONG:
MINUS POUNDS

New Door

Two years after receiving my diabetes diagnosis, I found myself reflecting on the experiences and improvements resulting from my changed eating patterns and exercise. First, the positive.

I was down to 216 pounds, 24 pounds less than two years ago. My diet was much healthier and very enjoyable. Fermented foods contributed greatly to my overall health, and resistant starches had remedied a few persistent problems with sleep and digestion. Two A1C tests, in September and December of 2015, indicated blood sugar levels of less than 7 where it stayed for 6 months (to remind, that means well-controlled diabetes).

However, even though there was a lot to celebrate, I wasn't where I wanted to be.

First and foremost, I wasn't satisfied with the speed of improvement. Twenty four pounds weight loss over two years is only a pound a month. Not overly convincing, especially when you consider how easy it is to gain a few of them back during the holidays or winter time when physical activity often decreases. Unfortunately, weight gain often goes hand in hand with increased A1C scores.

Actually, that was exactly what happened a year before, in the winter of 2014-2015 when my weight slowly crept back up. Now once again I gained a few pounds, I felt sleepy after mealtime, and my quality of sleep suffered.

These are subtle signs many diabetics learn to recognize. Sure enough, despite those two encouraging tests earlier, my A1C level jumped to 7.3 in March of 2016. Needless to say, this was frustrating.

Don't get me wrong, I didn't dismiss my accomplishments. It's just that my goals were a bit higher than merely well-controlled diabetes and a bit less weight. I wanted my weight to move from "obese" to "normal," yet my current 216 pounds were still in the obesity range. I wanted my A1C to go under 6 indicating diabetes in remission and giving me a chance to get off medication. In light of these aspirations, my results were far from satisfactory. My progress up until this point felt like I was laying a foundation. My next step was still unclear to me though.

As often happens, the door opened when I was ready to walk through it.

For a good while, my online research was showing sites claiming miracle recipes for reversing diabetes. As any person with an ounce of a common sense would, I was ignoring them.

However, in an attempt to remain open-minded and thorough in my research, I did glance at some of them. Unfortunately, they were largely a collection of miraculous promises to be revealed "in just a moment..." but first listen to this, read that, and of course pay this "very low fee" to find out that cure "that government and doctors hide from you." Or watch a video with the same promises, that never ends, can't be paused or fast-forwarded, and probably comes to that same "low fee" – can't say for sure, never watched those till the end. And "watch this before it gets deleted," and "the secret that was hidden from you for decades..." You get the drift. After a while though, I noticed some sites mentioning diabetes reversal that looked different and referred to a respected organization, Newcastle University. After researching the links to make sure they were legitimate, I started reading.

As I read through the description of the method and looked at the studies, it became clear to me that this was my next step and possibly a real breakthrough. Newcastle University's pioneering study showed encouraging results in reversing Type 2 diabetes in individuals who had lived with the diagnosis for up to four years, and in many cases longer. I have read the reports of multiple studies that followed, confirming the results, detailing the approach and fine-tuning the steps to take. Many people followed the method and reported inspiring results on various forums. Their stories had the air of authenticity and a lot of convincing details. The science made sense, too. Most encouraging, it looked simple (not necessarily easy, mind you) and doable without getting a degree in medical science.

The idea was fairly straightforward. See for yourself:

Normally, depending on your age, weight and level of activity, to maintain your weight you need to consume from 2000 to 2500 calories daily. That's your total daily energy expenditure (TDEE); you can check yours at one of the online calculators, like http://mytdee.com/. So, for five days of the week, eat just that, trying not to exceed the norm but not being overly strict about exact calories or (to a degree) composition of your food. For the remaining two non-consecutive days, eat 600 calories a day (500 for women). This is the general premise of the method. How's that for simplicity?

Of course, there is more thinking that goes into this, but that's the major idea. It's important also to understand the philosophy, if you will, behind the method of Intermittent Fasting (this is what this approach is called). It will help us understand our physical reactions and how to interpret them.

Why It Works

Fair warning: the description here is, of course, a simplification. You can go as deep as you wish into the intricacies of our metabolism and immensely complicated details of the biological, hormonal and chemical processes occurring in our body, and there still will be miles to go. I, however, assume that, within the framework of this book, it's an "engineering approximation" that we are after – a level of understanding that allows us to chart our course without becoming professional researchers in a medical field. I'll refer those who are eager to go deeper into theory to The Obesity Code by Dr. Jason Fung and The Fast Diet by Dr. Michael Mosley linked in the Resources.

It's not merely a lack of calories that promotes weight loss. Just as important is re-awakening our natural mechanisms for maintaining a healthy weight and body composition. Our bodies were not built at a time when fast food establishments and vending machines surrounded us like bees surround honey. Nor were there refrigerators and freezers to hold excess food at the ready, supermarket shelves full of cans, bags and boxes with anything we can or can't think of, always there and always lucratively looking. Our bodies learned long ago to function under much tougher conditions where the constant search for food dictated the optimal ways to preserve and expend energy. Feast-famine cycles commanded our bodies to store energy when food was aplenty, and use it up when food was lacking. Moreover, the expenditure of energy was strategic: At the first indication the food supply was getting low the body produced extra energy, to enable the increased range to hunt or gather. That makes total sense – if within our usual search radius there is no mammoth to kill, root to dig, or fruit to gather, we need to go further afield, and our body obediently serves up the required energy. It is only much later, in the famine stage, if the food doesn't become available after the extensive wait, that the body gets scared into starvation mode and starts saving each and every ounce of energy by making us feel tired so we don't move. During normal times our body alternated between fed and fasted state; our hormonal system that regulates energy uptake, storage and expenditure is built for such alternation.

This leads us to two logical steps.

First is an explanation of how we got fat when modern life interrupted this natural way of dealing with the historic vagaries of the food supply by making it freely available at all times. An endless feast stage is not what our body understands. It's trained to store energy when energy is supplied, and it does just that. It stores and stores and we get bigger and bigger. The natural defense mechanisms that signal us to stop eating (satiety hormones), are weakened by increased intake if sugar and refined carbohydrates. The famine never comes, and the stored energy never gets used. On top of that, by various reasons (of which the food industry's promotional effort is somewhat to blame) we were conditioned to think that hunger is something to be immediately extinguished or better yet, not allowed to occur at all. Somehow we've become accustomed to the idea that we need to eat so often that we furnish our day with frequent meals and snacks in-between to a degree probably never seen in history. Rarely do we go for an hour or two with nothing to chew or sip on. And if, gods of satiety forbid, we do feel a pang of hunger, it amounts to full blown anxiety attack – "I feel peckish, we need to find something to eat ASAP, where is the closest food establishment?" – and when we locate one, we shovel down another enormous portion of fries with gravy and muffin with coffee full of cream and sugar, and pack some donuts to go because who knows when we will get the next chance, maybe more than, perish the thought, two hours from now??

Fed state is characterized by elevated insulin; fasted state lowers insulin level. Uninterrupted fed state leads to constantly elevated insulin levels, and insulin commands the body to store fat. Worse yet, in an attempt to restore the status quo our body responds to the constantly elevated insulin level by increasing insulin resistance. In turn, the insulin level increases once again to overcome the resistance and keep blood sugar down. Recognize the vicious cycle in the making? Sure enough, these two duke it out behind the curtain for years, unseen and unheard, until the pancreas' ability to produce ever-increasing quantities of insulin is exhausted; that's when our blood sugar shoots up and we get diagnosed with pre- or full blown diabetes. Yet the signs of slowly rising insulin resistance manifest themselves before that if you know where to look for them. If you eat frequently, feel hungry without a snack every couple hours, crave sweets, slowly gain weight (especially around the abdomen) – in all likeliness the two forces are battling behind the scene and you are on your way to heightened insulin resistance and, eventually, diabetes.

Second step, of course, is how to go about re-training, or rather re-awakening our body's natural way of regulating normal energy inflows and expenditures. If we can find the line between making our body burn fat to support our food search on one side, and scaring it into starvation mode on the other – we will accomplish our goal. We will make ourselves function just as we were designed to; storing enough energy to find the next food supply, use it up in the process of finding that source and repeat this cycle naturally and effortlessly. We want to make our body a)feel the need for food, b)realize that it's not coming on that first touch of hunger, c)supply us with energy to increase our reach – and then reward it with just enough food for it to be satisfied that we are not about to starve. Restoration of this natural cycle coupled with brief periods of fasting sends the body into its natural fat-burning mode in which it uses its internal storage without attempts to store and preserve each and every crumb. The message we generate to the body is "you are doing the right thing, you have enough energy to find the next source of food, and it's coming; there is no need to get scared, continue burning fat and we will be just fine." It's not unlike training your pet by rewarding it for the right response.

Insulin is produced in response to food intake. Short-term fasting changes the hormone production patterns and levels to facilitate weight loss. It increases insulin sensitivity (double yay for diabetics!) and lowers insulin – this helps with fat burning since heightened insulin levels prevent the body from burning fat and promote fat storage. It also increases Human Growth Hormone (HGH) by as much as 5 times – that promotes fat loss and muscle gain. Finally, it increases production of noradrenaline, fat burning hormone.

Thus, this fat-burning mode requires a few simple steps:

1 Reacquainting ourselves with a healthy feel of light hunger and restoring our tolerance of it.
2 Training our body to give us an energy influx in response to that hunger.
3 Rewarding it by supplying the food soon enough, to create a positive feedback loop.
4 Structuring it all in a way that is easy, not too restrictive, and positive.

I can't stress this 4th point strongly enough. This is exactly where and why most diets fail.

They make us miserable.

They are unsustainable in the long run (just for how long are you going to tolerate being miserable?), and when they inevitably end, we return to our previous way of living and eating – and of course, looking and feeling. In this regard, you can think of this particular approach as a way of life rather than a diet. A way of life that is natural for us, easy and enjoyable – thus, sustainable. Also, by its very essence this is a pattern of eating rather than a diet.

Now is a good time to discuss a few variations of this methodology. Intermittent Fasting (IF) comes in a few different flavors. The one I described above is known as "5/2" and dictates that a small amount of food is taken over roughly 36 hours – a day and two nights twice a week, while eating normally the remaining 5 days.

Another version is almost the same but comes to merely 24 hours between full meals instead of 36. That means you have your last full meal in the evening and another – the next evening, filling the time between them with that lessened calorie intake. It's obviously easier to do and just as obviously somewhat less effective. Personally, I decided to keep it as a fallback option in case the 36 hours proves too difficult to do. That never came to be so I never used it. It still has its use, however. First, it can be effective during maintenance mode – something we will discuss later on. Second, it might be useful for a lightened additional fasting day. Again, we will get to it in the **First Month** section.

One more variation is "every other day." The name is pretty self-explanatory (as is another known name for it, "Alternate day fasting"); you eat normally today, fast tomorrow, eat normally again, and so on. Trying it on mentally and reading the accounts on the Internet, I came to the conclusion that it would have been a bit too stressful. This felt to me as one of those lifestyles that were prone to make you miserable when stretched over a long time. I did accept that there were folks who could do it routinely and stay happy; I just didn't believe I would have been one of them. I also accepted that my view on this could change down the road as my body learned to function differently. That remained to be seen. For the time being, I went with more moderate approach.

One more very intriguing modification is known as "16/8." Eat up to your normal calorific count every day, but do it within an 8 hour window, leaving 16 hours with no food at all. If you have 8 hours of sleep, have another 8 hours with no food and you are there. Break them down however you want – 4 hours after wake-up and 4 before going to sleep, or 6 and 2, or 2 and 6 – just make sure that you do not eat for 16 hours straight. This must be one of the easier ways to do it, with the only exception being some unfortunate social or work schedule on some particular day. At the beginning, however, I wanted to avoid any "every day" commitment and go with something that allowed me to forget about "dieting" for the most of the time. For that reason, I put it in the drawer together with the "24 hours" version to use later.

Then there was a version where you would eat 800 calories a day – every day. This one I shot down on the spot. No way, no how was I going to turn my life into every day's craving. I didn't even discuss that with my inner self.

There are some more variations but you get the idea. There is also this interesting idea of occasionally skipping a meal when you can – too busy, just not hungry enough etc. Just skip it and go on as normal until the next one. Mostly intended for generally lean folks rather than those who need to lose a lot of weight, it's still a nice weapon in arsenal for the most of us.

Thus, the decision was to start with the 5/2 version as the easiest to handle and very promising at that. The idea of always having "tomorrow to eat as usual" appealed to me. It sounded the least likely to make my life miserable; it was flexible and offered freedom for manoeuvre, and it just felt right.

Upon completion of sixth month I had enough experience with a few versions summarized in the Maintenance Mode section.

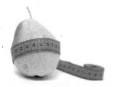

BEFORE JUMPING INTO PRACTICAL STEPS,
LET ME CITE ONE QUOTE NICELY AND CONCISELY
SUMMARIZING WHAT WE DISCUSSED:

Excessive insulin causes obesity.

When you eat, insulin goes up and your body stores energy. When you don't eat, insulin goes down and your body takes stored energy and uses it. Storing energy (sugar and fat) is the function of insulin.

When you have excessive insulin — higher than normal amounts and for much longer times than normal — your body becomes resistant to the effects of this hormone and produces even more insulin. It's a vicious cycle — and it doesn't matter what you do; exercise, diet. Too much insulin and you get fat.

So, how are we getting too much insulin?

Snacking.

We have an "eat all the time" mentality. In 1977, we were eating white bread and jam — which raises insulin levels — but we weren't snacking all the time. And we weren't obese.

In the last several decades, the number of times we eat in a day has gotten substantially higher. We've gone from three meals a day: breakfast, lunch and dinner, to six: breakfast, snack, lunch, snack, dinner, snack. We are stimulating insulin all the time, keeping it constantly high.

How do we bring our insulin down?
First, avoid foods that excessively stimulate insulin. Like, sugar and refined grains. That, we (as a society) have accepted.

But we also need to think about meal timing. We need periods of time when we aren't eating, so insulin can go down, leaving our bodies in energy burning mode. If we leave more time between meals — and, therefore, burning energy — we will lose weight.

So, fasting.
Yes. By fasting, we get our insulin levels low and we get rid of the resistance. Fasting, by dramatically lowering insulin, acts to lower the body's set weight.

Dr. Jason Fung, author of *The Obesity Code*.

Hunger in Practice

Before I began this eating pattern, I had to understand how to be comfortable with hunger. This is, I suppose, your major concern at the beginning, as it was for me. We are so un-used to feel hungry and so conditioned to prevent hunger that most of us are scared of it before we even have a chance to experience it. Our lack of experience dealing with hunger leaves us with very little knowledge of it (and unknown scares us), so some practical aspects of it come as a surprise.

The main misconception and the one that makes it so scary is this: as the first pangs of hunger come, we assume that they are going to build up and become stronger and stronger. Naturally, if they feel unpleasant and uncomfortable at the very beginning, just how painful are they going to become as food deprivation progresses? We expect them to become stronger and stronger, until they become unbearable, catastrophic, horrifying, oh boy, where is that food, need to get me some before I collapse in spasms ... whew.

In reality, that's nothing but unfounded fear. Nothing like that happens. Hunger, when ignored, goes away. Plain and simple. Let me repeat: hunger does not build up, does not grow stronger – it just goes away.

If there is anything astonishing about this, it's that it surprises us. More than likely, you have experienced this phenomena at some point in the past. You were busy with something, felt the first impulse to eat, got distracted by whatever you were doing and simply forgot about that impulse. Quite possibly, it returned much later, when you were done with your work, and you felt ravenous – but you did go for a few hours after that first twinge, and never collapsed or suffered any odious consequences. More than that, you were likely quite productive while completing the task that had you preoccupied.

Yet, under normal circumstances, we consider hunger unacceptable and go to great lengths to prevent it. When you consider that it comes in waves and doesn't escalate, you realize that, to paraphrase old saying, "the only thing about hunger to fear is fear itself." And that's just the first, though important, realization. Second, and just as crucial for our purposes, is this: hunger is a sign that things are starting to work the way we'd like them to. It's a first step in the chain of events we want to develop. It triggers the whole chain, and as such, it's something to **celebrate**, not to fear!

With all that in mind, let's talk about practical steps you can take to deal with hunger on your fast day.

First and the most effective weapon in your arsenal: drink. No, leave that hope at the door; wine and whiskey won't do. Neither will beer, milk or sugary sodas. Coffee will. So will tea, water, water with lemon, with cucumber, with or without ice, cold or hot. Coffee, of course, will be black and tea will be without milk or sugar. You will be amazed how drinks quell the hunger. You are likely to find that hot drinks quash it the most effectively. Hot water with lemon is my personal favorite – it's amazing how a large cup of that drink, simple as a rake and taking all of 5 seconds to prepare (OK, after water is boiled), supresses your appetite. Just drop a slice of lemon into a cup of the hot water, squeeze it a little and your drink is ready.

Second and somewhat unexpected (to me at least): delay your first meal as much as you can. Our body deals with hunger more easily in the morning as opposed to the late afternoon. Use it to your advantage by pushing your breakfast (on a fasting day) as late into the day as you can. By doing this, you achieve multiple goals. One is obvious: you shorten the remainder of the day to consume your allocated 500/600 calories. You also concentrate them in the evening, so it's easier to go through that time of the day when we often feel most peckish. Next, by consuming them closer to sleep time you avoid attempting to sleep while hungry. Last, but not least – by adding hours from your wake-up time to your first meal you increase the fasting time when you go with no food at all. Remember we spoke about launching that chain of reactions by awakening hunger? This increase of the fasting window is your first and most effective step in doing just that. If you had your last meal on the day before, let's say at 8 PM and your breakfast at 8 AM, then normally you'd have a twelve hours fast. You also have twelve hours ahead of you to live on 500/600 calories. Can you push your breakfast to 11 AM? You just made it a fifteen hour fast and have just nine hours to survive on those calories. And if you managed to wait till 1 PM? Seventeen hour fast and merely seven hours to endure limited calories. Importantly, it's at this time of fasting after the night sleep that production of Human Growth Hormone increases multifold.

The third one is fairly obvious – stay busy. Do whatever you can that requires your attention, keeps you distracted and helps hours fly. One very important thing about your fasting day is not to feel miserable, and there is no reason for that unless you chose to amplify any fleeting sign of discomfort by focusing on it. If it's a work day, it's easy to get preoccupied – things to do come naturally. If it's a weekend, there are home chores, a good book, a nice walk, an event to attend (not a food-related one, mind you), gardening – go wild and find nice ways to keep busy. The key word is "nice" – do something you enjoy doing.

Fourth and somewhat unexpected again – exercise. You would think that on a day with limited food intake you would need to preserve energy. In fact, just the opposite is true. Your body feels good exerting itself. It doesn't have to be some elaborate program. Just do something simple and enjoyable for the beginning (we will talk more about more pointed exercise programs on the fasting days later on, but on your first fasting days just try to stay active and enjoy it). Walk, cycle, do some push-ups, dumbbells, do some yoga or Pilates – anything that you like. Do that for just as long as you enjoy it. Have another hot drink after you have finished. Oh, and keep a room-temperature drink handy while exercising, and sip it generously to stay hydrated. We are going to have entire section on physical activity, so for the moment I'll leave it at that.

Most of all, and I can't stress this enough: adopt this grateful attitude toward hunger. Anticipate it eagerly; look forward to experiencing it as a sign that you have launched the process of weight loss. Appreciate the pang of hunger followed by its retreat as a signal from your body: got it, we are on our way to health and great physical shape!

There are some more steps to take, and I am going to go over them in the next section describing preparations for the first fasting day.

Preliminary Decisions

Don't think for a second that it was all too clear from the start that a fasting day was going to be a piece of cake or even doable at all. You see, the first thing you are told when diagnosed with diabetes is to eat frequently and regularly. Every three hours, in fact. In light of everything I know now, I really question this advice. Making your pancreas work non-stop, having insulin levels raised constantly? Adding more of what has caused the problem in the first place? That, however, is an official position and being a new patient, who are you to doubt it? After a couple years of following it, I seemed to be a walking confirmation that the advice was correct. If I had no meal within a 3-4 hours window, I felt some kind of abdominal distress, bordering on pain. In reality, I probably simply cultivated and reinforced this reaction by following the advice. To avoid that distress, I made sure that in situations away from food I always had some snack within easy reach. Thus, the first signs of uneasiness were met with that snack, and most often I wouldn't even let those signs appear, going just by a clock. So, that was a real concern – how was I going to handle long periods with no food at all? Wouldn't those pains kill the whole plan right at the starting line? That was simply something to try and see.

Preparing for my first fast day, I thought about how I was going to organize it. There are some practical details to decide upon, for instance:

- What exactly am I going to eat?
- How many meals a day am I going to have and at what time?
- What my schedule for the day is going to look like?

Thinking of what to eat, I faced two decisions to make: my food composition and exact products to use. Food category-wise, it was fairly obvious. I wanted this day to be mostly proteins and vegetables. The idea was simple: proteins keep you feeling full for a longer time, and vegetables help with fiber content, which is needed on high protein days. Meanwhile, the fats have a bit too high a calorie count for a fasting day, and the sweets and carbs would lead to food cravings. In fact, I have observed, communicating with other fasters: those who ate fruit had more difficulties dealing with hunger. With that in mind, I started surfing the Internet for corresponding recipes and calorie counts. This is where I realized that I disagree with the commonly accepted approach to this matter.

Try to read any book on this kind of diet, and you will find a practically uniform view: to make your diet easy and pleasant, you need to introduce a lot of variety, have multi-component dishes presenting varying tastes, making your food entertaining. Your regimen should not be boring or monotonous. Sounds obvious, right? I beg to differ. You see, this angle is applicable to long-term diets where you would have to endure long periods of eating with certain limitations. For those diets it's a reasonable approach – assuming, of course, the diet itself is a sensible one. In this particular case, though, we are talking about one fasting day you need to undergo, and the next day you are back to your regular diet. And on this fasting day you need to eat relatively little and wait for that next day. Wouldn't it be logical to avoid excessive focus on the food during this day? Don't we try to keep ourselves busy and distracted on this day, to be focused on something other than food? Now think of a (relatively) complicated dish – wouldn't you be fixated on preparing it? If it's a multi-ingredient dish, wouldn't you be faced with putting it together, surfing through your kitchen cupboards and refrigerator shelves, taking in all the sights and smells? When we eat something really intriguing, is our first impulse to stop eating it after a small portion or is it to grab another? Finally, when a dish we prepare requires multi-step preparation, won't the process itself fire up our appetite?

All this convinced me that my approach should be different. On the fasting day my food should be tasty, yet simple and familiar. It should be exceedingly easy and quick to prepare, or even require no preparation at all. It shouldn't trigger imagination or invoke curiosity – hence the "familiar" requirement. It should be a food easy not to think about. At the very least, all this is true for the beginning stages of this diet – first few weeks, maybe a couple months, until it becomes a routine and we are fully in control.

What is tasty, simple and easy to prepare? Why, eggs of course. Boiled, fried, scrambled – love them in any shape or form. Protein – check. Quick – check. Easy – check.

What else? How about chicken breast? Half of a medium-sized one with the skin removed is about 140 calories. Got some fish or meat leftovers from the previous day? Look up the calorie count and grab a piece of a corresponding size. Got a can of salmon? Perfect – protein goodness with all the ease of opening the can! Got some legumes cooked with any spices of your choosing? Few things can beat that for a fasting day. Add a piece of a carrot, a couple of leafy greens, cherry tomato or a fork-full of sauerkraut. There – a simple and tasty meal taking next to zero attention to prepare, and filling you with protein and fiber. And to finish off the day, a cup of kefir made from full-fat milk is exactly 150 calories.

Having planned the day's menu with those bits and pieces, I thought of the meals' schedule. My first impulse was to go for 4 portions, 150 calories each. I felt that more meals spread out over the day will make it easier. While it might be true for some, further experimentation showed that three meals a day, 150 – 300 – 150 calories, worked out better for me. It allowed for longer periods without food (remember, that's an important part of the fat-burning mode), and it allowed for a longer period of satiation following the 300 calorie portion. For the moment though I decided to have a breakfast between 11 AM and Noon (instead of my usual 7 – 7:30), and go as long as I could before the next meal, with the last one consumed at 9 PM.

Lastly, I planned what to do throughout the day, to stay hydrated, busy and active. I felt it was important to plan the day in advance in order to just follow the plan without much room for thinking about what to do. While it ceased to be a factor later on, it was a good idea for the first day (and even first couple weeks) of fasting. It was also a good idea to do it on the weekend the first time. While it seems a bit counter-intuitive to the idea of staying busy, the first time you fast you want to be in full control of your time and your actions. Starting a new experience, such as fasting, during an already busy day could increase your levels of anxiety and discomfort.

In order to be ready for the morning without food, I had my last meal of the day before close to 9 PM, and made sure it was mostly protein, to keep me going as long as possible.

Finally, before I describe the first day, I would like to discuss one more thing. Any kind of changes in your lifestyle are much easier to make when your family takes part in it. Chances of success are much higher as well. I was lucky enough in this regard: my wife wanted to shed some pounds as well, and also became just as interested in this approach. Iryna was at 178 pounds at that point and saw 160-165 as her target. Actually, she dreamt of even lower numbers but didn't think them achievable. In fact, even those 160 seemed a bit unrealistic to her at that point. Also, she was taking a diuretic to control her blood pressure, just as I was. Thus, we decided to do it together.

So, here was my starting point:

Weight: 216 pounds;

Waist: 42"

BMI: 31 (obesity territory)

Fat Percentage: 32.6% (obesity territory)

First Day

To suppress the usual "OK, breakfast time!" signal from the body in the morning, I started the day with a glass of water with potato starch (you of course remember this one from the chapter about resistant starches). Some morning Internet surfing, news, checking e-mails and doing small house chores took me to 9 AM. Interestingly enough, hunger didn't really manifest itself – I felt pleasantly light and energetic. The feeling was kind of "I could eat something and enjoy it, but I have no problem going without food either." Thirty minutes later, emptiness in the stomach felt a bit more pronounced. A cup of hot water with lemon at this point was a good idea; it made me feel full for about an hour. Spending time at my computer, writing a couple of documents and answering some e-mails filled this hour, and by 10:30 I felt the first hunger impulse. That was the moment I waited for with some trepidation. Will it be bearable or will those stomach pains put an inglorious end to my plans right at the starting line?

A cup of strong black coffee was my third drink of the morning. When I say "strong," you better believe it. In our household, coffee is made the traditional way in a jezva – a Turkish pot designed specifically for this purpose.

Once again, the hot drink worked just fine. With a huge sense of relief I felt the hunger retreating – no pains at all. Neither did I experience a lack of energy. Just the opposite, in fact – I felt a strong desire to move, walk fast, put some effort into something. I used this energy influx to do some push-ups and stretches, and it felt fantastic. This experience was consistent with the theory of fasting – having no food at the usual time, my body apparently decided to give me some oomph to go further afield and find that mammoth.

Around 11:30 I finally rewarded myself with a fried egg and a strip of bacon, topped by a piece of a carrot and a leaf of lettuce. I expected myself to wolf it all down in a couple of huge bites. Just the opposite happened. I ate it in small pieces, slower than usual and enjoying each bite. The taste felt greatly enhanced. In fact, I found that my usual amount of salt felt a bit too intense, and made a mental note to decrease it a bit next time. Bacon, of which I was and am a fan, was full of fatty, smoked, crispy goodness. Even the lettuce was sweet and tasty – and traditionally I've been quite indifferent to leafy greens. Finally, even though this meal was about 1/4 of my usual breakfast, I didn't feel empty. Neither did I feel full; rather, it was an agreeable compromise. I heard many times (and dismissed it as nonsense) that you need to leave the table with light sense of hunger. This was the first time when I suspected there was something to it. It wasn't an unpleasant feeling at all. Still, it remained to see how long it would sustain me.

Thirty minutes later we went for a walk. We walked noticeably faster than usual. It wasn't on purpose; we just followed what felt right and enjoyable. With the level of energy we had, brisk walking felt good and highly gratifying. It was a great indication that so far we were on the right path. One thing we realized quickly was that we'd better plan the walk so that there was a washroom in close proximity, as the body was flushing water at a much faster rate. We will return to this in the separate section, as this is a part of a broader phenomenon.

At 1:30 PM we returned home and around 2 PM had our next cup of hot water with lemon. This drink was quickly proving to be a real saving grace. Easy to prepare and amazingly helpful with making you feel full for a while, it remains on our menu for both fasting and non-fasting days. We decided to have our remaining meals at 3 and 6 PM, with a cup of kefir at 9.

150 calories at 3 PM felt every bit as good as the morning portion. A cup of tea and some water sustained me for the next couple of hours, but around 5 o'clock I started feeling pangs of hunger much stronger than those in the morning. Once again, my experience was consistent with the theory of fasting: mornings were much easier to handle. It made sense to increase the time between waking and breakfast, allocating more food in the afternoon. Still, the pattern continued: as long as I could distract myself, hunger would recede without escalating.

The 6 PM meal felt a bit on a smallish side. My body was obviously untrained for such a scant food supply. Still, I was satisfied with my ability to handle it. I assumed that if I could survive the very first day with no pains and with no cravings strong enough to render me incapable of coping, it could only get better later on as my body would get used to new regime. That proved to be true beyond belief, but we will get to it in good time.

Some more hot drinks between 6 and 9 PM, and finally a cup of kefir to end the day. I made myself drink it slowly, and I have to say, as much as I enjoy every cup of this heavenly drink, that particular one was absolutely spectacular. Smooth, fizzy, with a perfect sour bite... wait for me, be right back.

Being able to fall asleep with a mostly empty stomach was another concern. It proved to be easy though. The accomplishment and anticipation of tomorrow's morning weigh-in indication followed by the full-scale breakfast created a lot of positive sentiment.

Next Day

Next morning brought two surprises, both pleasant.

The first was about expectations for the morning hunger and feeling extremely anxious about having breakfast as soon as possible. You would think that the next morning after the fasting day you should feel like eating a horse in one bite. This proved to be completely wrong. Not only did we wake up well-rested and feeling good, we didn't feel starved. In fact, we had our breakfast about 30 minutes later than we normally would, and felt perfectly fine about it. It's not that we didn't want to eat – no, there was this normal morning feeling of being ready to put some fuel in the tank. There was also, however, this newly added sense of being in control. The sense of being secure even without an immediate food supply. Starvation anxiety went away. Hunger was no longer a scary beast. A single day of fasting gave us this completely changed attitude toward hunger – instead of being frightened by it we now perceived it as a welcome sign of the success of this approach. Instead of being an enemy to fight off, it turned into our ally. Instead of feeling relieved that the fasting day was behind us, we discussed the exciting perspective of the next one!

Breakfast tasted amazing. Mind you, it was our usual breakfast, but our taste buds seemed to develop heightened sensitivity. Against all expectations, we didn't eat any more than on any other day. In fact, we found ourselves being satiated a tad earlier than usual. Our normal portions felt slightly excessive. So we decided to try and cut the portion a bit starting the next day. This decision worked well for our non-fasting days allowing additional decreases of the overall calorie intake. Curiously, that was absolutely effortless, natural, and happened seemingly by itself. It was as if the body, upon being reminded how to function properly, happily remembered it and began fixing the imbalances right away, starting with the amount of food it demanded. And that was the outcome of just one fasting day? That was highly encouraging.

The second surprise was my morning weigh-in. I expected some drop, of course, that was the whole point of fasting. But what I saw exceeded all my hopes. Three pounds in one day!

Now, the meaning of this number requires a separate section. The one I promised when mentioned how we had to make sure the bathroom was somewhere nearby throughout the fasting day.

Water Weight

It's important to understand the role of water during weight loss drive. Fat is not all we lose when we slim down and it's not what we gain when we finish our weight loss regime. Here is what happens when we burn fat, through fasting or otherwise. Again, the explanation below is somewhat simplified, so if you are a medical doctor, try not to cringe. We are trying to chart our course, not to learn all the scientific facts of the subject.

As we consume carbohydrates, our body turns them into energy storage in the form of glycogen. When there is enough glycogen stored, the body puts the over-supply in fat. Think of it as short-term fuel and long-term fuel. A significant detail is that glycogen requires water to be stored, and a lot of it – each gram of glycogen needs about 3-4 grams of water! What happens when we start a weight loss regime? In the initial stage, our body depletes glycogen stores and releases water in the process. With that ratio, no wonder our first day (week, and even month) results look so impressive!

You can see now where all the water output on our fasting day came from. There wasn't a sufficient energy intake, so when we went for a walk our bodies had to use glycogen to keep us going. The depletion of glycogen released the water used to store it, hence the need to plan your routes with bathroom proximity in mind.

That explains the larger drops at the beginning of our weight loss attempts. It also explains why we inevitably regain a few pounds when we finish our diet – the body replenishes glycogen stores and retains more water to do that.

While it might be disappointing to realize that there is not much (if at all) fat eliminated in those first pounds, there is no bad news in this. First of all, this is simply a necessary first step, as the body gets to burn long-term fuel after it goes through the short-term one. Second, the opposite side of that coin is those frightening weight increases that we might observe sometimes after a big party with a lot of food, particularly carbs, sweets and alcohol. While they might trigger panic in you ("Oh boy, did I really gain 5 pounds in one night??"), in reality it's mostly that same water weight (plus of course the food still making its way through your intestines). A lot of energy has been taken in, stored as glycogen, and 3-4 times as much water had to be retained for that. It's only if you continue collecting without spending that excesses of short-term fuel will be converted into long-term fuel – fat.

Understanding that, you will no longer be frightened by those sudden bounces in your weight, inevitable when you have a few days heavy on carbs. Nor will you be discouraged when your pace of weight loss inevitably slows down after the initial stage – burning actual fat is accompanied by much more modest amount of water.

Do avoid the temptation to fight back by drinking less water. As counter-intuitive as it is, drinking more and not letting yourself feel thirsty helps with water expulsion; faced with lack of water intake a body tries to retain what it has.

To stop being disheartened by the water weight fluctuations, think of yourself as a car with a tank full of fuel. Registering your technical parameters, you may record your weight with an empty tank and it will look a tad more favorable. The reality though is that you do need that fuel, so consider these fluctuations a normal cycle of burning it and refilling the tank. Just make the distinction between "weight with empty tank" and "weight when fully refuelled."

First Week

Two days later we repeated the same routine, this time having breakfast at 1 PM. Additional hours before breakfast were filled by an additional cup of Tulsi tea, some more physical exercise and work. This is when we both noticed one more effect of fasting – intensified mental clarity. Actually, we experienced it on our first day as well but we have assigned it to being especially attentive to every minute thing.

Less time between the first meal and sleep made this day even easier than the first one. We ate the same food, avoiding being needlessly creative. It once again helped to keep our focus off food. Most of the patterns and sensations repeated themselves – the same bursts of energy leading to a faster pace during our walks, and the same ease of handling the hunger pangs. One noticeable difference was in the intensity of those pangs. They became much duller – we could still feel them but they were almost an afterthought, kind of a weak signal that didn't even try hard to get your attention. It was as though the body, getting a message that screaming for food didn't achieve the result, stopped screaming and learned to do without. At the same time, it quickly learned that it wasn't about to starve; after all, some food did appear as it waited so it could just as well start consuming some of its internal storage to sustain the wait.

The morning after the second day of fasting showed me a 1.8 pound drop. Expectedly smaller than the first day result, it was still fairly sizeable. I probably still wasn't losing a lot of fat, but things were going in the right direction. Most of all, it was still easy, exciting and promising. None of the worst fears materialized – no pains, no insomnia, and no adverse body reactions of any kind.

Once again, my next day's food consumption was normal; there was no need to compensate for the fast by overeating. Once again, I couldn't help but notice how amazing everything tasted. The very process of eating became more deliberate and every morsel became more enjoyable.

As we finished the first week, I was about 4 1/2 pounds lighter. Iryna was not far behind at 2 1/2 pounds. I started tracking my weight every morning after the fasting day on a sheet of paper, writing down the actual weight and the progress from the last one. I'm going to detour from the storyline for a second to talk about the subject of weighing oneself. In this regard, I once again found myself differing from the commonly accepted advice.

Most often you can read everywhere the suggestion to avoid weighing yourself daily. The idea behind this recommendation is to ignore the daily fluctuations that can be influenced by many factors. Instead, you are supposed to focus on the bigger picture and track your progress by, say, a weekly measurement. The approach that works best for me is different. I wanted to track those fluctuations and understand them as much as possible. They opened an empirical window of sorts into the inner workings of my body. More so, I weighed myself twice a day, before going to sleep and upon waking up. This helped me understand my water retention patterns. I started seeing which foods influence it, how the sleep impacts my weight, what happened after physically exhausting vs. lazy day etc. etc. Those are all little details that create a better understanding of your body and make you more sensitive to the fine changes in your regimen. And about that possible discouraging effect? I resolved it by simply re-framing my goals and expectations for these frequent measurements. I didn't do them solely to track my progress – I mostly did them to study my body's responses to my experiments. I also formulated clearly that it's a weekly and especially monthly progress that is indicative of my real progress, and whatever happens in-between is mostly interesting for those educational purposes.

This approach gave me a better understanding of my optimal sleep times, and timing and composition of the last meal of the day. My average overnight weight change (which of course reflected water retention) was 2 pounds. Most times when I went to sleep between 10 and 11 PM, not only did I sleep the best and wake up well rested but I also saw the best overnight weight loss, between 2 and 2.5 pounds. Delaying going to bed beyond 11 usually made falling asleep more difficult, decreased sleep quality and resulted in less overnight loss bracket, 1 to 1.5 pounds. The last meal was best taken between 8 and 9 PM, and a cup of kefir or 100-150 g of cream-cheese seemed to work best, maybe with a few walnuts, almonds or a handful of crunchy roasted chickpeas. Adding fruit, however, resulted in more water retention.

Your particular discoveries of course can and probably will be different. That being said, your view on the frequency of weighing yourself can be different too; you may or may not be as curious about all these details as I am, and that's completely fine. I just want to present another approach so you have your choices better laid out.

First Month

Not knowing what kind of results would be realistic, my secret goal, as a sign of great success, was 200 pounds. While still overweight, it would be an impressive number of pounds to lose – or so I thought at the time. What I did not expect was that the very first month would put me within spitting distance of that goal. I lost almost 13 pounds by the end of the first month. Here is a scan of my sheet with the breakdown of the results after each fasting day, loss from the previous one and running total.

march 19 - 213 (-3)   216
211.2 (-1.8)
209.2 (-2.0)
208.2 (-1.0)
207.2 (-1.0)
Apr 6   206 (-1.2) -10 overall
204.8 (-1.2)
204 (-0.8)
Apr 19   203.4 (-0.6) = 13

WEIGHT LOSS PROGRESS, MONTH 1

My belt went to the third hole. Energy was overflowing. No weight loss plateau, no boredom from the eating plan. The results were all positive. Iryna lost 8 pounds over this month, so we were both on track toward our respective targets, and moved fast.

We spoke a lot about how the whole method turned out to be very different from what we expected. No matter how many accounts I've read of other fasters with similar results, the prospects of staying hungry for the whole day, twice a week, seemed a bit intimidating. At the very least, it promised to be a bit of a struggle – the question remained how much of a struggle it was going to be. Chances are, if you never fasted, that's exactly how you view it while read these pages. That proved to be totally incorrect, and boy, did we feel happy about that!

There were a few more things we noticed during that month. Interestingly enough, fasting days stopped being something unusual or drastically different from any other day. We found ourselves taking longish walks with no worry at all that we might get hungry. The only word I can use here to describe this feeling is liberating. Remember how I was afraid to find myself with no food at hand every 3-4 hours? Now that leash was severed. The only thing I needed to remember was to have some water handy, but that's advisable for anyone, fast or not.

The most striking instance of this new perception came when during a long walk we discussed the dinner menu for the evening and whether we needed to buy some groceries on our way back – and suddenly we remembered that this was a fasting day! When we realized that in the middle of the fast we plain and simple had forgotten that we fasted today, it became abundantly clear to us that our fasting routine became just that – absolute routine, fully integrated into our lives and demanding no effort.

An interesting pattern emerged in our physical state. We felt better on fasting days than we did on non-fasting ones. Any signs of being tired would appear sooner on normal eating days than during a fasting day. Any kind of uneasy feeling in the stomach would manifest itself only on eating days as well. So much so that we started joking about food being optional and possibly even harmful to human bodies.

Speaking of the normal eating days, we haven't really kept to a strict regimen of counting calories. Instead, we just got the general sense of various foods' caloric value and did an approximate count of our typical breakfast and other meals. Putting on a sheet of paper our most frequently consumed foods and their calorie counts, we quickly assembled a list of separate foods and various combinations. This list grew with each new food we added, but it still fit on a single page. Throughout the week we did a running total by adding each meal's count and monitoring the sum at the end of the day. Week-long evaluations of our most typical meals in this fashion gave us a pretty good general sense of such tallies and, aside from the occasional search for and weighing of something new in our menu, we mostly stopped paying attention to it. Being attuned to your food intake and body's reactions, you gain a solid sense of your caloric intake for the day. To prevent the possibility of eventual creeping carelessness, we did infrequent (say, once a month) checks of our day's consumption, making sure that our old habit of overeating didn't find its way through the backdoor. This approach helped us to keep honest without the restrictions and tediousness that come with constant counting and measuring.

Speaking of a calorie count, I want to mention one more habit that fails many of us. I call it "**MINDLESS MUNCHING** ." Sit in front of the TV, put a bowl of peanuts in front of you and see how long it will take for them to disappear. Tasty, crunchy, and you don't even worry much about them since you know they are good for you, right? Now I will wait for you to check how many calories one cup of those peanuts brought with it.

. . .

Have you regained consciousness? Yes, you read it right; your eyes didn't deceive you. Over 800 calories. In one cup. A full meal consumed without even noticing and, I bet, without cutting down the calories in other meals that day. And this same dynamic applies to many snacks we munch on mindlessly, while enjoying our favorite leisure pastime. Often it's not even something we fully enjoy eating – it starts off this way but then becomes just an automatic motion of grabbing yet another handful without noticing. Meanwhile, nuts are one of the best snacks you can think of – compact, chock full of energy and nutritional value – IF you consciously make them a part of your daily intake and remember that they are not to be eaten mindlessly.

Now, how about that movie theater popcorn with butter? I can sense the resentment starting to boil in you – yes, you know it's outrageously high in calories and hopelessly low in nutrients, but that's not the point of eating it, is it? When you want to relax and enjoy something without thinking of how unhealthy it is, the last thing you want to hear is, well, how unhealthy it is. And I am right there with you (even though popcorn is not my vice). Just go ahead and enjoy it, but make sure that you compensate by cutting out something else, or adjusting the calorie count for the next day. Nothing bad is going to happen – as long as it's an episode and not a habit. Start doing this regularly and you will cause real harm. But the thing is, you won't even want to. Not if you modify your lifestyle as this book describes. We will get to this in our **Second Month** section.

Meanwhile, speaking of snacks, we almost completely banned them, even on normal eating days. This was in line with the general idea of training our bodies to work with full sized meals and deal with between-meals periods without additional food intake. Now if we did take some nuts or fruit with us during the walk, it was only when we had an unusually long time to go before the next meal. However, we never made this a strict limitation on ourselves; if we ran into a blackberry bush while walking around the lake, we never denied ourselves the ripe berries during their glorious season. The philosophy is simple: enjoying life and not restricting food unnecessarily (well, eating sugar by spoons would be a notable exception).

On the third week we came up with another interesting twist – **"LIGHTENED ADDITIONAL FASTING DAY."** Completing our fast on Wednesday, we discussed the scheduling of the next one. Two candidates were Friday and Sunday, both days looked good for that. Friday, however, would have been separated from today by just one day, which might have been a bit too soon. We just didn't know whether it would feel like too much too fast, but we were curious to find out. The idea we generated was to assign Sunday as a scheduled fasting day, and come Friday – to start it as a fasting day but keep it light, so to speak, not too strict and with self-given permission to deviate at any moment. In practice it meant that we were going to go with the flow of the moment; if such frequent fasting proved to be difficult on Friday, we would add some food or even switch to normal eating altogether. Maybe it was going to end up with 800 calories, maybe 1200 – in any case it would be a "fasting light." We assumed that such an attitude would make it fun and very easy. Knowing that as an extra day we could stop it at any time without breaking the regimen should aid in handling this fasting day so soon after the previous one. And, if that day went well (ended up being a full fast mode that is), it would be a Sunday's turn to be treated as an additional day, with the same mindset.

You probably have guessed by now how it went down. Yep, both Friday and Sunday ended up being fasting days. Knowing that there was a way back at any moment made it especially easy; the realization that we effortlessly pushed our weight loss mode one step further in such a playful manner made it especially pleasant. We've repeated this experience later on when we felt like it, without specific plans, going just by the mood.

If you feel like adding another day to your two, you may want to consider making it a lighter one in another way – make it 16/8 day or 24 hours fast day, as we described earlier when discussed IF variations. This will make it fun, easy and won't overstretch your willingness to fast.

Second Month

The rate of slimming down slowed during the second month, which was not surprising at all in light of what we know about water weight. Still, it was a respectable 7 pounds:

march 19 - 213 (-3)   216
          211.2 (-1.8)
          209.2 (-2.0)
          208.2 (-1.0)
          207.2 (-1.0)
Apr 6   206 (-1.2) -10 overall
          204.8 (-1.2)
          204 (-0.8)
Apr 19   203.4 (-0.6) -13
Apr 25   201.8 (-2.6)
    27   199.8 (-2.0) -16.2
          199.0 (-0.8)
May 12   198.4 (-0.6)
          197.6 (-0.8
May 19   195.6 (-2) -20.4

WEIGHT LOSS PROGRESS, MONTH 2.

Most of all, I was happy to leave behind the former goal of 200 pounds. What was perceived as a floor, became a ceiling now. Obviously, that target was too modest; this new approach was capable of giving me more. Also, there was an annual visit to the doctor's office around that time. My blood pressure normalized greatly – 117 over 72. My waist size dropped to 40 inches; I was at the last hole of my belt and even that felt a tad too loose, so I made a 5th hole in it. My BMI dropped to 28.1; that was no longer obese, but in the overweight category. Iryna's results were just as nice, with a 5 pound loss now at 165. That was the upper limit of the range she wanted to achieve. Considering the ease with which we both came to this point, our ambitions were significantly higher now – or is it lower when we speak of weight targets? 160 looked achievable, and she started setting her sights on 155 pounds – something she wouldn't even say out loud a month or two ago. For myself, I decided that if I could reach 190, I would consider every pound after that a bonus. Seriously, it would have been a 26 lb. drop, and I would be around 20 years back in the time machine – that's how long ago I weighed 190! If I could achieve more than that, great. If not – I would be happy with that.

And why wouldn't we be optimistic? Unlike many diets that grow more and more difficult with time, this regime was becoming easier. Actually it's not even the right word since, somewhat surprisingly, it wasn't hard to begin with. It became an indistinguishable part of our weekly routine, unobstructive and unnoticeable.

Also, at the end of the third month I was going to have my next A1C- indicating how weight loss had affected my blood sugar levels, so I had a significant milestone ahead.

Speaking of new experiences and discoveries, we did have some. Remember I mentioned how tasty everything was on the next day after our very first fast? This sensation became constant, throughout all of our normal eating days. It was as though our sense of taste intensified. Everything we enjoyed before we enjoyed many times as much now. That cultured butter on toasted buckwheat bread was absolutely heavenly. Kefir-based cream-cheese with garlic, black pepper and herbs... OK, I'll shut up now. This filled our non-eating days with the excitement, looking forward to amazingly tasty things tomorrow.

An unexpected discovery was that while the taste of healthy foods became intensified and more pleasurable, the taste of unhealthy foods became less appealing. The starkest example of that would be sweets. Many of those treats we used to like became almost unbearably sweet. You are familiar already with this effect; we discussed this same kind of experience in the part devoted to cutting down and replacing sugary foods. Now this experience multiplied in intensity and spread to some other foods.

Do you like chocolate cake? So do I. In one of the local stores there was the chocolate cake of chocolate cakes. King of chocolate cakes. They don't get any chocolatier. It was called Chocolate Eruption, and it was a massive bomb. Real chocolate cream, rich and smooth; chocolate layers of different colors and varying consistency with pieces of hard chocolate to provide a crunch. Did I mention it was also full of chocolate?

At the beginning of our new weight loss regime we put two large pieces of it aside, to reward ourselves for some significant achievement should such occasion present itself. For two months we felt a great temptation walking past the baking section in that store and seeing that cake on display. We waited patiently for the time when we would deserve the prize. Finally, in mid-May, that moment came. They were rather large pieces, mind you – the reward should be generous and leave you fully satisfied, not craving for more. We ate it all... and were surprised by just how incredibly sweet it was, beyond the sweetness that would have been pleasant. We were cured; walking past that section has become, well... a piece of cake!

This tendency spread to fast foods and eventually to sweet treats and ice-cream. Now we take a different approach to these items, and indulge in small portions of high quality treats. Organic bakery small eclairs from hand-milled flour filled with hazelnut buttercream vs. largish standard issue supermarket eclairs with whipped cream – the choice was clear. If we wanted an ice-cream, we preferred real stuff and not a low fat creation with an artificial sweetener.

Even some long-standing staples in our menu underwent some changes. For instance, we used to make a sweet version of our cream-cheese by mixing it with some jam. Now we preferred to mix some berries in it with no sugar added. Strawberry, raspberry, blueberry, blackberry – some of them crushed and some left whole – everything was delicious. Try any of the berries you like and enjoy new combinations of the taste. Or, if you want something more ice-creamy, mix those berries with crème fraiche (again, our self-made probiotic version), and put it in a freezer for a short while; add some vanilla extract if you want to imitate that flavor. Adventurous? Mix in some cinnamon. And most of all, there is absolutely no sugar needed not after a few weeks of getting your taste buds retrained and especially after a few weeks of fasting. You are already familiar with many dessert ideas without additional sweetening, so I'll just address you to that part of the book here.

The same change occurred regarding the quantity of food. We just needed less of it now to feel full. Maybe it happened because when your body is at a lower weight it requires fewer calories to maintain it. Maybe a higher density of nutrients found in healthy food caused satiation more quickly – quality wins over quantity. In any case, that was another good development reassuring us that the change was sustainable. Actually, in one way we found this to be a challenge; we had so many great dishes to eat that we simply didn't have enough mealtimes to try them all. They formed a long line waiting for their turn to be cooked and consumed. Things that used to be taken out of a freezer weekly now could spend a month or more in the freezer. It was a good trade off: our food expenses dropped noticeably while the quality of what we ate became exceptional. In an interesting dichotomy, on one hand, there was a decreased need for or want of food. On the other hand, there was an increased curiosity for new foods and a newfound enjoyment of foods that were of good quality.

During this second month we also switched our fasting day breakdown to three meals: 150, 300 and 150 calories. First mealtime would often come around 2 or even 3 PM, never earlier than 1. The second would occur at 5-6 PM, easily sustaining us until the last meal, around 8-9 PM. We found this regime the easiest and most natural for us.

Third Month

Speaking of dichotomies, you probably noticed by now this interesting contradiction. On one side, I talk about how routine and unnoticeable fasting days have become. On another, I emphasize the excitement we experienced during this entire time. How to reconcile these opposite states of mind?

Have you ever caught yourself dreaming of some great accomplishment while not focusing too much, if at all, on the efforts needed to achieve it? You are not alone. In fact, I don't think there is a single person on this planet that hasn't. In some way, this pattern of eating has been a good match to such a dream as it accomplished just that. Effort was minimal and non-intrusive while the results were grand and exciting. If at the beginning of our fasting we naturally concentrated on our sensations and experiences during non-eating days, this novelty quickly wore off and they turned into routine. At the same time, general changes in our bodies continued, and with them excitement of the achievements grew and new realizations developed.

First about the numbers though. On June 19 I hit 189 pounds, losing 27 overall:

WEIGHT LOSS PROGRESS, MONTH 3

That kept a pace of 7 pounds a month – the speed of weight loss didn't drop compared to the second month. This was true for Iryna as well – she lost another 5 pounds and sat at 160, the target she thought too optimistic three months ago. That was most pleasing; with the exception of the first month and its disproportional water weight, my body slimmed down steadily with no signs of a dreaded plateau. My belt became useless, and I had to buy a new one. The BMI indicated 27.1. Finally, there was that impatiently anticipated A1C test at the end of June. It indicated 6.3.

Needless to say, I was on cloud nine. The drop of 0.9% over the course of 3 months was nothing to sneeze at. I moved from poorly controlled diabetes into the so-called "pre-diabetic range." The threshold of 6 was within spitting distance. Even if there were no other signs of health greatly improving, this alone would have been a fantastic indication.

And there were many a sign. First, I was no longer experiencing intestinal distress. While I used to experience some kind of uneasiness or stomach-aches regularly, which didn't seem to be attributed to a particular food or combination of foods, such cases ceased completely. Small aches and pains in the joints, which we usually attribute to aging, disappeared. Swelling of the ankles and wrists, particularly on a hot day, also ceased. My Time Machine worked!

And speaking of those long walks – our favorite 10 km loop around the lake was probably the best indicator of how much our health has improved. For years, we used to make that loop in 2 hours and 20 minutes of pure walking time – that is, after we subtracted time spent near a blackberry bush, in a washroom or on a bench with a spectacular view. We used to dislike parts of the route with any incline. Also, on the last few kilometers we would slow down somewhat and feel noticeably tired. Finally, upon coming home after such a walk we were done with any kind of physical activity for the day, we just felt tired enough.

By the end of our third month of IF, we noticed changes in the speed with which we walked the route, and we didn't even notice the incline anymore. We didn't slow down during the final stretch, nor did we feel spent when we completed the walk, often going for another walk later in the day.

We found a nice way to incorporate some treats into our routine. If there was a wonderful bakery with some tempting pastry near our walking route, we would have that pastry with a cup of coffee before hitting the road. Walking right after that helped burn those sweet calories before they did their usual thing. Guilty pleasure without guilt – try to beat that!

Fourth Month

At the height of the summer season, the challenge is to keep up with the abundance of amazing fruit and berries. Cherries, blueberries, raspberries, strawberries, plums, figs, apples, you name it. We expected that such an influx of carbohydrates could slow down our progress. Our actual results, though, proved to be almost the same as before: 6 pounds more (or is it less?) for me and 4 for Iryna.

June 27   187 (-1.5) -29 overall
June 29   A1C 6.3
          186.4 (-0.6)
July 7   185.6 (-0.d)
          185.0 (-0.6)
          184.4 (-0.6)
July 14   183.4 (-1.0)
    19 - 183 (-0.4) 4 months,
                 - 33 overall

WEIGHT LOSS PROGRESS, MONTH 4

Sitting now at 183, I lost 33 pounds in 4 month and 4 inches off my waist which was at 38" now. My BMI at 26.3 was within reach of the normal weight range. Based on healthy BMI recommendations, I was within 15-20 pounds of my ideal weight. This didn't feel too difficult anymore – my ambitions were now greater than my previous "every pound under 190 is a bonus." I had seven such bonuses already under my belt (literally!) and saw no reason to stop there. Iryna, at 156 pounds, started talking about 150 and below – whatever happened to that former timid "165 would be so nice."

You of course have heard many times this well-known statement that the signal "I am full" from our body comes with some delay after we have eaten enough. This lag often leads to over-eating. By this time we have developed a fine-tuned sensitivity to this moment. It's difficult to describe; you don't really feel full yet, but somehow you know the moment when it's enough. This sense differs from the "I could burst at seams" or "I can't possibly stuff anymore in myself." It comes way earlier than anything of the "full" kind and it's unmistakable. Your connection with your body becomes stronger and its messages clearer.

Fifth Month

Ten days later, with an increasing onslaught of ripening fruit, we faced a decision. Plums from our backyard and figs and apples from our friends' trees could go spoiled while we limited our consumption on fasting days. I found myself at 180.4 pounds while Iryna still remained at 156. So we decided to experiment with another variation of Intermittent Fasting for a week or two. 16/8, where you could eat normally every day within an 8 hour window while fasting for 16 hours, seemed a perfect fit for this time. We would have our last meal (why, a cup of kefir of course) at 9 PM, and postpone our breakfast till 1 PM. Since late breakfast was quite easy for us to do now, we thought it was the easiest way to proceed, while not letting all that gorgeous fruit go to waste. If necessary, we could always add one day of usual fast to the week of 16/8 to keep the pace intact. So, starting Aug 1st we switched to this regime for a couple of weeks to see how it went.

As expected, mornings were not difficult, even though we now did this breakfast delay every day and not just twice a week. A glass of water with potato starch, a cup of coffee or tea, hot water with lemon – all the tried and true methods of keeping the hunger at bay worked just as reliably. Also, as 1 PM rolled around, we didn't hit the fridge with rage. We just started preparing our usual breakfast around that time so the actual meal would come at about 1:30. Neither did we inhale it quickly – despite 16+ hours of complete daily fasting, we were able to eat in a measured manner. This deliberate way of eating became quite pronounced during these months, whether on fasting or eating days.

Having 8 hours to eat as usual, we haven't used permission to consume full daily allocation of the calories. It was as if we simply cut one meal out of our ration. We had another full-sized meal at around 6 and a cup of kefir at 9. That was quite enough to keep us fully satisfied.

In a week after beginning this regime the surprise came. Believe it or not, we missed our fasting days! We enjoyed them, loved how they made us feel – light, energetic, in full control. This once again confirmed that our new way of life was sustainable; it's easy to do what you enjoy doing.

We decided to modify our regime to accommodate one fast a week. The following two weeks were a combined 16/8 and 6/1 mode, where we had our 500/600 calories one day a week and ate within an 8 hour window for the remaining six days. That worked out amazingly well. The weight loss during six days of the 16/8 pattern was slow and gradual, without the dives that we experienced on fasting days. However, there were no after-fast bounces either, so the fasting day would take us to the new lows faster. You will see two such plunges at the Aug 7 and 14 in the screenshot below. The effect overall was just as impressive – despite all that fruit onslaught, the month ended with a seven pound loss, which marked an increase of the pace vs. previous:

19 - 183 (-0.4) 4 months,
         - 33 overall
July 27 112 (-1.0)
   181.6 (-0.4)
July 30 180.4. (-1.2) 38" waist
Aug 1 - 16/8 beginning

Aug 7 179 (-1.4)
   178.6 (-0.4)
   178.0 (-0.6)
Aug 14 177.0 (-1.0)
Aug 17 176.4 (-0.6) 5 months.
        - 40 overall

WEIGHT LOSS PROGRESS, MONTH 5

Forty pounds over five months came to an average eight pound a month, or two a week – a very respectable steady rate that by the weight loss standards is widely considered healthy and sustainable. With BMI at 25.3 I was within spitting distance from a healthy range which starts (or is it "ends?") at 24.9. Just 10 pounds separated me now from my target weight which was looking very reachable over the next couple months. I started this sixth month with firm determination to achieve 170 pounds, 165 in the seventh month and then possibly over-shoot it a little so that the inevitable bounce at the end of the weight loss drive would stabilize around 165 and never go above 170.

Not to lose the track of Iryna's accomplishments, she once again shed 5 pounds finishing the month at 152. That constituted a 26 pounds loss overall for her.

Sixth Month

We have kept the 16/8 regime for most days this month, and we decided to add some experiments to it. At this point I thought we were ready to try a 24-hour long fast. There were two variations of it I wanted to test. One would have ended with a full-sized meal, while another – with a 500/600 calories portion. My interest in them was triggered by reading the studies that claimed the maximum effect of fasting has been achieved in the window between 16 and 24 hours. I also started formulating the strategy for the maintenance regime, which we will discuss shortly, and wanted to gauge my body's response to a 24 hour fast, to see whether it was a good fit for that regime.

Probably, not the smallest of the reasons was pure curiosity – it was interesting for me to evaluate just how far my newly gained control over hunger went. At the beginning of this whole fasting adventure even a few hours seemed to present a challenge, but I thought I became capable of much better management since then.

This assumption proved entirely correct, for both of us. Not only were we able to fast for a full 24 hours, the very sensations of hunger changed greatly. At the beginning of our weight loss drive we labeled it as "pangs" and felt it as an unpleasant state bordering on pain. It used to be something to overcome, to get distracted from and to fight off. Not at this point though – now instead of a distressing sensation we simply felt awareness that our stomachs were empty. It had no negative emotional connotation; it was simply an acknowledgement. If anything, it was even mildly pleasant. It's a somewhat difficult feeling to put in words – a mix of sense of accomplishment, satisfaction of being in control, sense of good things happening to your body. Add a good energy level throughout the day and you get the picture. Actually, "good energy" might be an understatement; for the first time ever we completed our traditional 10 km loop around the lake in two hours, shaving a good twenty minutes off our usual time while maintaining conversation and not losing our breath.

Ending our 24 hour fast with 500/600 calories turned out to be not any more difficult than having a full-sized meal. If anything, a full meal felt a bit too heavy. The morning after showed a sizeable weight loss, advancing us quickly to our goal. I have marked those days on the record sheet. Sixth month ended with me at 170 pounds, for the 46 pound loss since the beginning of the Intermittent Fasting regimen and 70 pounds from the diagnosis. (See image on page 216)

BMI at 24.4 was now in the normal range.

Iryna finished this month at 147 pounds, shedding another 5 and reaching a 31 pound loss overall, with her BMI standing now at 25.2 – still slightly overweight.

175.8 (-0.6)
Aug 31 174.6 (-1.2) − 24H
174.2 (-0.4)
173 (-1.2) − 24H
172.4 (-0.6)
171.8 (-0.6)
171.2 (-0.6)
170.8 (-0.4)
Sept 1 170.0 (-0.8) 6 months,
− 46 overall

WEIGHT LOSS PROGRESS, MONTH 6

Seventh Month

At this point, however, our plans have changed once again. A good plan shouldn't be rigid and must be adaptable as new data alters the view. Here is what happened.

Our biggest achievements were in our dramatically decreasing need for drugs to control our conditions. At this point with our family doctor's blessing we both stopped taking diuretics to control our blood pressure. For a few weeks, per doc's instructions, we took our blood pressure several times a day – first thing in the morning, after an exercise session, and before going to sleep. It stayed normal without the help of drugs for the first time in many years. Finally, my next A1C test came back at 6, which was within spitting distance of the healthy range. My dose of Metformin went down to minimal. A correctly fed body healed and needed less to no help from the medicine. All good, right? Yes, but...

As soon as we stopped diuretics, our weight went up – about 4 pounds for Iryna and 6 for me. All the water pushed out by the medication returned, raising the scale indication. Sure, it was just water, not fat, but it changed our numbers nonetheless. You don't answer the question about your weight with "oh, it's 170 but 5 of them is just water," do you? So now we needed to eliminate this bounce, and then continue our weight loss drive toward the target.

I didn't find much about this situation in my research. How large a bounce is normal and expected when you stop taking diuretics? How long should it take for the body to expel this retained water and return to the weight before the bounce? What are the "mechanics" behind this? Reading all I could find and speaking with a few friends from the medical field led me to the following, which is not set in stone, so I share it with an open mind to changes:

- While there is no exact numbers or per cents to evaluate the bounce size, 4-6 pounds is nothing to be alarmed about;
- Strength and dose of your particular medication influence this number; so does your overall weight;
- It takes your body a couple of weeks to gradually realize that the crutch it relied on to expel the water is no longer there, and to start working without dependence on it;
- It takes about two weeks to a month to return to your weight – **providing your body can control blood pressure and water retention on its own.**

If it all works and you can maintain your normal blood pressure without a diuretic, it's a fantastic development. Even the least invasive medications with minimal side effects present an intrusion in many processes and functions. Stopping these medications restores the natural balance to your body. It all went according to the new plan. A month later, we returned to our pre-bounce weight numbers, this time with no help from a drug and with blood pressure firmly within the normal range. Needless to say, our family doctor approved. To quote, "You guys are now officially off the medication. Do take measurements periodically to make sure everything is fine, better to stay vigilant... but overall, congrats! This is what we love seeing in our patients."

With this somewhat unexpected delay, we continued our regimen.

Eighth Month

As close as 5 pounds from my goal, I started evaluating where I was in regards to my physical shape. Two factors made me think I needed to make some additional correction to my lifestyle. One was waist to height ratio achieved – at a 37 inch waist and 5 ft. 10 in. height I sat at 0.53, while a healthy ratio demands under 0.50. Second, obviously connected, was purely visual: I could see some fat rolls on my stomach. My ambitions have been raised once again; I've decided to continue the weight loss regime with no specific time or weight in mind, focusing more on this particular indicator – waist, where the abdominal fat resides, clinging to the internal organs and causing maximum damage. To concentrate the effort on this target I decided to increase the role of exercise, paying particular attention to resistance training. Up to this point I was exercising to make sure that my muscles are preserved during my weight loss drive; now I wanted to gain muscle mass to help with eliminating these remaining pounds of fat around my waist and achieving a lean body composition. Instead of doing a set of resistance exercises for each major muscle group and completing a circuit for the day, I started doing multiple sets for a particular group in one day, targeting different groups one after the other and applying much more effort to develop each of them. You will see the details of my physical regimen in the Exercise section. Here, I'd like to remark on the same familiar motive that manifested itself earlier in my attitude toward fasting and repeated now in regards to the exercise: I loved how it made me feel, both during and afterwards. I started missing it on the days when for this or that reason I didn't do any, and I did everything possible to incorporate at least some bits and pieces. Another score for the sustainability of the new lifestyle!

With the Intermittent Fasting routine and the increased role of exercise, by the end of the eighth month the long-standing goal that seemed so ambitious was achieved:

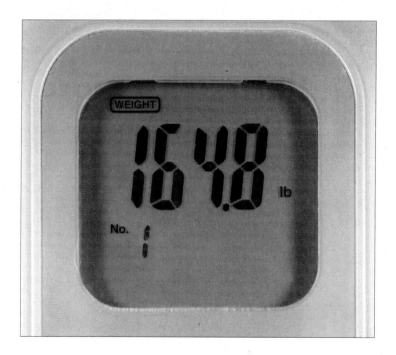

My waist was now at 36 inches, 8 inches slimmer. Body fat at 23.2% and BMI at 23.7 all indicated a healthy range. Total weight loss from the day of diabetes diagnosis amounted to 75 pounds; about 50 of them were lost during the Intermittent Fasting regimen over last eight months.

Iryna's results: 141 pounds, for the 37 pounds loss over 8 months, with her waist circumference at 30 inches, about 3.5 inches slimmer.

It's difficult to describe the euphoric sense of accomplishment we experienced. The weight, look, state of health and physical shape that we could only dream of turned out to be realistic and achievable in a shorter time than we could imagine. The process turned out to be highly exciting and required no great sacrifice or suffering.

Now it was time to switch to the Maintenance Mode which I will describe in details. But first, let's talk about the exercise regime.

Exercise

Purposeful physical activity is an integral part of the weight loss regime, as well as an equally important part of staying healthy. The benefit of exercise, particularly for diabetics, is very real and demonstrated in endless studies. Physical activity significantly improves glycaemic response, lowers A1C and reduces visceral fat (as always, you'll find links to the corresponding studies in the Resources section). It also plays well with fasting – somewhat counter-intuitively, exercise feels right on fasting days and amplifies the positive effects.

Being lean and fit, looking and feeling your best, while not making exercise a major part of your day sounds like a reasonable objective. I will assume that those are your goals, as are mine. If you are a bodybuilder or a competitive athlete, you probably are better served with different book.

Do you like the gym? Neither do I. I am not adverse to exercise; in fact, I like how I feel after a vigorous workout. I just want it to be more natural, convenient and less time-consuming than typical gym routines and settings dictate. In fact, I want my workout to be over in the time it typically takes to *drive* to the gym.

Do I need special motivation for working out? Honestly, no. Remember our discussion of the motivation in the beginning of this book? I said back then:

"I have difficulty understanding the very concept of needing a strong motivation to improve your health. Doesn't a chance to prevent or reverse diabetes, look and feel your best constitute the strongest possible motivator of all? If such a prospect doesn't inspire you, nothing I could say will."

I feel the same way about a need for motivation for working out. I look at my "before" photo, and the burning desire not to look like this ever again is enough to motivate me. I read my initial A1C report, and the resolute determination to beat this death sentence is enough to motivate me. There are my kids with their careers just starting out, and there is my grandson with his whole life ahead of him – isn't a wish to see it all unfolding enough to motivate me? Would any standard excuse, like "the weather isn't good" or "I need new sneakers," stop you if you formulated your goals this way?

... Didn't think so. So, let's drop all this "special motivation" nonsense and just do what it takes to stay healthy. Your "before" photo, your bloodwork sheet and photos of your family is all incentive you need. If it's not enough, no clever tricks or crafty speeches will inspire you. Just one practical tip that might come handy: no matter how lethargic you feel, as soon as you warm up your body feels good and enjoys the movement. So, when you feel heavy, sleepy and unwilling to work out, just stop ruminating and give exercise a chance; it will get easier and feel better in just a few minutes and you will be glad you dragged your bottom off that couch. The feel of slightly complaining muscles after the workout is not at all unpleasant either. Also, just exercise for a week or two and see how good it feels to have more energy and a sense of a body protected by an armor of newly-found muscle.

Main principles that governed my approach to the workout were pretty much in line with those that I used creating my diet. It must be sustainable in the long run to become a part of my lifestyle. A routine that you start, run for a few weeks only to drop it and return to a sedentary way of life is not much different from another fad diet, and just as useless, if not outright harmful for your health. I wanted it to be simple, fun and consume as little time as possible. I wasn't about to spend hours in gym or torture myself with exercise routines that would make me groan. At the same time I realized that a certain effort must be applied for a workout to be effective. Without pushing one's body to do what feels uncomfortable there is little chance it would become stronger. Thus the challenge was to find a fine line between what was effective and what did not make me miserable.

The Routines

Let us break this section in three parts: cardio, resistance training and flexibility exercises.

CARDIO

For the most part, I am not too enthusiastic about this kind of training. Folks that spend hours on cardio equipment in gyms in hope to shed pounds and improve their cardiovascular system have been misled. It plays its role in our undertaking, and it's an important role, but the way it should be done is different from the majority of time-wasting efforts promoted as health inducing holy grails. Let me quote the bestselling author and trainer of elite Special Operations forces Mark Lauren:

> It is a myth that doing prolonged steady state training – usually maintaining a target heart rate for 30 to 60 minutes – like aerobics or "cardio" is the best way to burn calories and achieve cardiovascular health. Ever plod along on a treadmill that tells you the number of calories burned? You might go 45 minutes before you hit 300 calories. Well, guess what? That's 300 total calories burned in that time, and not 300 calories above what your baseline metabolism would have burned anyway, even while at rest. That's the reason the exercise machine asks

your weight: To calculate your baseline metabolic rate. The average male burns 105 calories at rest in 45 minutes. Those 195 extra calories that the exercise actually burned – only 195 calories more than if you had been taking a nap – can be undone by half a plain bagel in half a minute. And aerobic exercise typically spurns your appetite enough to more than offset those few actual calories burned.

There is more to it of course, but I'll leave it to you to check out his book and arguments, as well as other skeptics regarding using traditional long low-intensity cardio exercises for the purpose of losing weight and multiple studies showing its low effectiveness.

That said, cardio exercises make their way in my regimen in three forms.

The first is simple **WALKING,** mostly for the purpose of lowering my blood sugar level. It's amazing just how effective a 30-40 minute walk is in getting your blood sugar under control. Studies show how an increase in daily step count correlates with a clinically significant reduction in waist circumference and BMI and decline in A1C. Upon taking blood sugar measurement before and after a stroll and seeing how rapidly it drops, I came to think of it as of taking my blood sugar outside and shooting it. I even used it to keep down the glycemic spike after a carb-rich meal (just don't take it as an encouragement to eat more of those and counter them with a walk, okay?) While not being a

---

*   *You Are Your Own Gym – The Bible Of Bodyweight Exercises For Men And Women*

huge calorie burner, walking works in many other ways to facilitate fat loss. Lowering your insulin (a fat-storing hormone) level is most important of them; so is the increase of lipoprotein lipase activity – that's the enzyme that lowers the amount of fat circulating in our blood vessels.

Do it outside as much as possible. I am fortunate to live in one of the nicest areas with an abundance of parks, beaches and lakes, all extremely walkable and providing a wide variety of enjoyable experiences. However, most urban settings do have parks and walking paths nearby; hopefully you have access to a few. Such walks are very relaxing; they allow you to shake off the stress of the day, so you get multiple benefits from one activity. Turning house errands into walks is often helpful – walk (or bike) to the store instead of driving where the distance is reasonable. I am not a fan of treadmills but if you have one and the weather is categorically forbidding, by all means use it. It's not necessary to push hard for speed; just try to walk as briskly as is comfortable. As your fitness and energy levels improve, you will want to walk faster – let this sense of the most suitable speed guide you. This effect will be especially noticeable as you slim down during your Intermittent Fasting regimen.

The second cardio workout I have built in my routines is what I call "**NO TIME WASTED**." It's simply an attempt to build some movement into the daily routine by combining it with activity that you would do anyway, just in a sedentary fashion. If there is a book or a magazine or a working document that you need to read, you can do so on a treadmill or a stationary bike, providing you have either. I do a lot of my reading on a stationary bike.

Then there is a TV. Since my family room doesn't accommodate sport equipment, I found a cheap way to incorporate it while keeping it, well, a family room rather than gym. I bought a cheap portable exercise bike, the kind that has no seat – it's just a small frame with pedals. Sitting in front of TV set, I plop this thing in front of my chair and by the time the show is over, I have anywhere from 30 minutes to an hour of additional sugar- and fat-burning added to my daily balance sheet. Not being enthusiastic about devoting time specifically to aerobic exercise, I'll gladly take it in parallel with something otherwise done in a physically inactive way. In their Fast Exercise book, Dr. Michael Mosley and Peta Bee remark:

> *"Simply by standing more, pacing around a bit more, taking the stairs, and walking when you can, you should burn through at least extra 350 calories a day."*

To put it in perspective, that's a pound of fat in 10 days (again, do not consider it permission to eat more!) Along with this concept also goes the idea of **fidgeting**, which we will investigate in the Resistance Training part.

The third and final way is also the most effective and intriguing. You may have noticed that stating my indifference to a cardio exercise I used the term "traditional long low-intensity." There is, however, a much more interesting and effective kind of exercise that can be done in a fraction of the time. I am talking about **HIGH INTENSITY INTERVAL TRAINING (HIIT)**– short bursts of intense activity with periods of rest in-between.

The effects of this method of exercising are so striking and so contradictory to what we have been told over our entire life that most have to read many studies, or better yet, try it themselves to believe it. In study after study, HIIT demonstrates a considerably better reduction in insulin resistance, A1C and body weight comparing to continuous training. Improvement of metabolic health is especially significant in those at risk of or with type 2 diabetes. It's particularly effective at burning fat, especially abdominal, or visceral, fat – the most important in determining your health. Amazingly and counter-intuitively, it also proves safe in individuals who seem to be at most risk with this type of exercise – those with a history of stroke or heart attack. Not entirely surprising and in full accord with the theme of this book, HIIT is also the natural rhythm of child play (without realizing it of course), and, as far as researchers can tell from studying isolated tribes leading primitive lives, that was the natural way for our ancestors to move. That alone can explain why our body responds to this kind of activity much better than it does to a traditional low intensity prolonged exercise.

Where does the secret of this near-miraculous way to exercise lie? It's probably in the so-called EPOC (Excess Post-Exercise Oxygen Consumption), or the after-burn effect, where you're burning more calories after the workout because your body has to recover from the intense all-out effort done anaerobically (with insufficient oxygen). To quote The Tabata Protocol website (more on this particular kind of HIIT follows),

"When you create an Oxygen Debt (read: heavy panting) your body has burned off all of the blood sugar (glycogen) it has and needs to replace all of that energy. It does this by burning fat. You don't want to try and burn fat WHILE you are exercising. You want to burn off CARBS as fuel when you are exercising."

From the previous sections you are well familiar with the concept of exhausting your glycogen resources to start burning fat during the Intermittent Fasting; we are now again in that same territory and it shouldn't be surprising at all that HIIT is so effective in conjunction with IF. I try to schedule my HIIT workout in the morning of the fasting day to achieve maximum combined effect. This way, the workout burns the glycogen, so in its absence any additional activity and even basal metabolism during the rest of the day feed off fat as much as practically possible.

You will find a variety of HIIT routines on the internet. My favorite is done on a stationary bike. Easy to alternate speeds, easy to regulate resistance level, it's ideally suited for rapid intensity changes prescribed by HIIT protocols. If you have an access to an elliptical, stair master, or rowing machine, they'll do as well; treadmills are trickier since they can't start and stop rapidly enough, you'd have to jump on and off of them, which might not be a very safe thing to do. You will also want to download an app for your phone or a tablet that provides a timer with sound alerts for the workout and rest times and round counts There are quite a few free aps for all devices, and most do basically the same thing, allowing you to use a standard protocol or customizable for tailored routines; just search for Tabata timer.

I tried a few protocols and eventually came to like two of them. The first is good for beginners that just get into HIIT. In its beginning form it consists of 15 rounds, each round consists of an 8 second workout and a 12 seconds rest. Before you shrug and say "That's all?" consider that in those 8 seconds you go all-out, giving all you've got to pedaling as fast as humanly possible. After the first round you will feel like you can do it in your sleep; a few rounds later you are not likely to be able to pedal at maximum speed through the entire 8 seconds, and by the end of the workout you won't believe how merely 5 minutes could have worn you out so much. Start with a minimal resistance setting; add some as your fitness improves, and eventually add a second 5-minute set. When you reach 20 minutes, this is all you need to do three times a week.

There is also a 30/90 variation, with 30 seconds workout and 90 seconds rest. And 15/10. And many more.

My favorite though is the classic **Tabata Protocol**, named after Japanese researcher Izumi Tabata, who conducted extensive research on HIIT in 1980s. This protocol is a default setting in many apps and dictates **20 seconds of all-out cycling followed by 10 seconds of low intensity cycling, 8 rounds for the whole of four minutes**. Seriously. That's all. Three times a week. Don't you love that?

If you never tried HIIT and just reading it makes you feel like you can do it without breaking a sweat, you are partially right – this kind of exercise doesn't make you sweat. It doesn't mean, however, that it's done effortlessly;

just the opposite is true. It's difficult to believe just how strenuous those measly 4 minutes can be when you do it right. You don't do HIIT monobuttockularly... okay, let's call it half-heartedly – a phony effort may fool a side observer but not your own body.

Before you start happily pedaling, a few important points:

- Don't do it more than three times a week. Overdoing it is not only pointless, it can be counter-productive.
- Warm up by gentle pedaling for two-three minutes; cool down after finishing the 8th round for two minutes. Cooldown is important, don't skip it.
- Start with 2 rounds if you are not fit and add 1 round a week until you reach 8.
- If you are not out of breath and seeing stars by the end of the last round, you are not giving it all you've got. Don't spare the effort; the whole point is in pushing yourself to the limit for a very brief time. It'll be over in just 4 minutes!

You will find a few more details pertaining to your particular case at the Tabata Protocol website linked in Resources section, but for the most part you just read the whole thing. I for one love both the brevity and simplicity of the exercise, and the ease with which it can be incorporated into any schedule.

The combination of HIIT, walking and additional movement intentionally added to an otherwise sedentary activity presents the perfect mixture of high and low intensity training for maximum effect.

RESISTANCE TRAINING

Gaining muscle mass, the most metabolically active tissue, is paramount to our fitness, metabolic responses and overall health. Just as with cardio, I see no need for using a gym and special equipment. Nor do I have any desire to go to a gym, for the same reasons as discussed earlier – time saving and convenience. Your own body weight is sufficient enough to do resistance training of any difficulty level and for any purpose, from general fitness to athlete performance. Common objects around us can be used for these exercises, some and minimal and inexpensive equipment completes all you might ever need.

I use two forms of resistance training, bodyweight training and fidgeting.

BODYWEIGHT TRAINING is familiar to most of us in the most popular exercises. The fact is that you can duplicate practically any exercise typically done with special equipment should you want to work on specific muscle groups. As far as I am concerned, one positive side of bodyweight exercises is less isolation; instead, it targets more muscle groups in a single exercise. This is more natural and holistic than the artificial isolation of a particular muscle achieved with specialized machines.

Not being or aspiring to be a fitness instructor, I'll just describe those exercises I do regularly and point you to a competent source for more details and drills.

Whether you just want to maintain fitness or seeking to develop large well-defined muscles, you'll have no trouble finding all kinds of routines on the Internet searching for 'bodyweight workout." For my purposes, the previously quoted and linked in Resources book by Mark Lauren is all I need and then some. Whichever you choose, I would like to encourage you to pay attention to the correct form of each and every exercise by carefully reading the descriptions and studying illustrations and videos freely available on the Internet, to make sure you protect your body from injuries and achieve maximum effect.

The routine below usually takes about 20-30 minutes. Depending on schedule and purposes, I either do the entire circuit on a single day with fewer sets or, more frequently, separate them by days targeting different muscle groups and doing more sets and repetitions. In either case, the whole workout never takes more than 30 minutes.

First thing in my arsenal is of course a push-up. It's difficult to overestimate this all-too-familiar exercise that targets many muscle groups. It has a few variations, and I try to do all of them in a single workout. I start with 'rocking chair" – slow deliberate movement forward and back pushing from your toes while in classic push-up position. It's done in both upper position (arms extended) and lower (arms bent in elbows). Next follows the classic push-up. I make sure I do it in a slow controlled manner while maintaining good shape – straight body with no arched back. Slight changes in the angle of your hands and distance between them changes the muscles on which the exercise is focused.

Then I do a Chinese push-up, also known as an inverted V or a pike push-up; in the downward-facing dog yoga position you either form a diamond with your thumbs and index fingers touching in front of you, or just keep your hands apart as usual (these variations hit your muscles under slightly different angles so you may want to alternate them from one workout to another), and do a push-up by bending your elbows and lowering your head, while keeping your back and legs as straight as possible and keeping your elbows from moving too much to the sides.

Next is a bit more dynamic version that targets the entire body. Dive Bomber starts with the same position as inverted V, while keeping your hands and feet slightly wider for better balance; when you lower your head toward the floor, drop your chest while moving your head forward and up, as if trying to slide under a bar. Straighten your arms pushing up, arch your back and look up. After reaching this position, reverse your entire motion by lowering your chest and head and push back with your arms to return to the starting position.

The final exercise in this series is a plank, targeting your core and back. The standard plank is done resting on your elbows and forearms. There are also many variations that add many other muscle groups, linked in Resources – not only do they create a whole class of exercise in its own league, but also introduce a fun variety that breaks the boredom of a routine.

Next in my routine is the curl, to target the biceps. I have a set of dumbbells which I use for this, and I do a free-standing version, not a sitting one with the elbow resting on a support. This way the entire body is involved in maintaining balance. The same holds true if I use dumbbells for a lift above the head, to exercise my shoulder muscles. I do a few sets alternating the arms and a few simultaneous curls with both hands.

If you have no dumbbells, no worry – there are a few ways to do this exercise without them. If your desk is sturdy enough, simply sit in your chair; put your hand under the desk, either making a fist or with open hand, and push against the desk upward. Simpler yet, do an isometric curl by using both of your hands – one in curl position pushing upward and another holding it down. Alternate hands to give one a biceps workout while another tenses a triceps. Finally, you can use a towel held by your leg at the floor while your arm stretches it in a curl position.

Next come the leg exercises. Large muscles in the lower body are especially important to develop and maintain. This circuit targets glutes, quads, hamstrings and calves.

First is an amazingly simple, fun and surprisingly difficult exercise. Stand on one leg, lift another slightly and close your eyes. That's all. Think it's easy? Use a stopwatch to see how long you can do it, and you'll likely to be shocked to find out just how brief your time is till you have to grab onto something or touch the floor with your other leg. Practice this pose to stand for up to one minute, and feel how your leg muscles tense in the process.

To exercise my quadriceps, I do classic squats. Glutes and hamstrings get worked as well. It's very important to make sure that your knee doesn't move beyond your toes as you lower your bottom to avoid hurting the knee joints. Just as with push-ups, small changes in the angle of your feet and distance between them redistributes the load between the muscles.

A wall squat is a static variation that makes it easier on your knees. Take a sitting position with your back against the wall, knees bent at 90 degrees and located straight above your ankles. Keep this pose for as long as you can as your thighs feel the burn. Sixty seconds is a great time to aim for at the beginning, but don't be discouraged if you can't do more than twenty the first time you try that. Do a few sets, letting your muscles rest and repeating the exercise.

Glutes and hamstrings get seriously loaded with the next two exercises. One is a simple extending your legs intermittently while lying on your stomach, arms along your sides. Make sure you don't push with your hands; instead, focus on squeezing your glutes as you lift the leg. Do a slow controlled movement with one leg a few times; as muscles start burning, switch to another. Alternate them for a few sets. When you gain strength, do a more difficult version – extending both legs, spread them to the sides and move back together slowly; this move will squeeze your glutes very effectively.

Another is a hip extension using a chair. Lie on your back, arms at your sides and your heels resting on a chair, knees bent at 90 degrees. Using only your legs, push your hips upward as high as you can. Your thighs should be in a straight line with your back. Hold this peak position for a two second contraction, squeezing your glutes. Then slowly lower yourself to the starting position. To increase the load, lift one leg upward and do the exercise with one leg only.

Lastly, I do a calf exercise by standing on a slightly elevated platform (a thick book will do; just make sure it's a phone book, not Dickens, okay?) so that only the ball of my foot is on the platform and my heel is in the air. Lowering my heel to stretch the calf muscles and pushing up, I repeat it on both feet, then switch to one alternating them, and finally varying the speed to finish the set.

The workout described above is a basic one, focusing on main muscle groups for complete training. You will have no troubles adding your favorite exercises to it. Keep it intense and short – this way you won't get bored and the benefit will be maximized.

Another way I incorporate some simple muscle-targeting exercise is **FIDGETING**. Not all of the movements we discuss below belong to pure resistance training, but many do and they all pursue the same purpose and fit into "using your own body" category, so to simplify the flow I put them all here.

Fidgeting has two purposes. One we discussed earlier – it's incorporating certain exercises in otherwise passive activity. My favorite example is doing calf raises, glute squeezes or partial squats while brushing your teeth. Isometric curls using both your arms while standing on a bus stop or waiting in line in the store is another. Sitting in the chair (which we unfortunately do a whole lot) opens up a huge realm of possibilities, believe it or not. Do a curl at your desk which we described earlier for your biceps; reverse the direction by placing your hands on the desk and pushing downward to exercise your triceps. Put your palms in front of you and push them together for exercising your pectorals. Push down into the floor for 5 seconds with your feet while sitting to blast your quads, glutes and hamstrings. Do calf rises. Squeeze and relax your stomach muscles. Raise your arms to the shoulder level and push against the imaginary walls at your sides, then in front of you; then raise them up and push against the pretend ceiling. Place your hand against the side of your head and try to push against the hand. Lock your fingers behind your head and push forward. Put your feet together and squeeze your ankles, then your knees.

I believe you are getting an idea and feeling just how creative you can be. In fact, I am doing them as I write this book. During any inactive time or a time taken by something requiring little attention and movement, it's easy to add some specific movement targeting inactive muscles – even if it's simply tensing and relaxing them slowly or in a quick succession. Granted, you are not likely to become a ripped athlete this way, but it's a fun way to add some movement and burn some additional calories. How much? It depends. While the number will vary widely depending on the type of activity, intensity and time, estimates can go as high as 300-350 calories a day. Most of the activity studied to come up with this number is done subconsciously by many people; others will benefit if do it deliberately. Among physical activities adding up to that caloric burn researchers list: standing periodically instead of sitting, stretching, shifting body weight between your feet, pacing whenever possible, walking around while speaking on the phone, tapping feet and wiggling legs, drumming fingers, shifting body position often while sitting, etc. Scientists called this kind of movements NEAT which stands for non-exercise activity thermogenesis.

Here are some curious numbers for you from the study done in Mayo Clinic in Minnesota. Subjects' energy expenditure was measured in various activities compared to control position (lying on their backs motionless).

- While sitting motionless, they burned 3.7% more calories than lying on their backs in the control condition.
- While sitting and fidgeting, they burned 54% more calories than the control.
- While standing motionless, they burned 13% more calories than the control.
- Standing while fidgeting burned 94% more calories than the control.
- Walking at 1mph burned 154% more calories than the control.
- Walking at 2mph burned 202% more calories than the control.
- Finally, walking 3mph burned 292% more calories than the control condition.

You will notice that the little isometric exercises I listed as fidgeting in the beginning are planned unlike largely subconscious movements researched in the studies. Together, they could add quite a lot, so if you are not a natural fidgeter, do try to introduce these intentionally. (You will do well trying to make these movements noiselessly, not to annoy people around you by endless tapping or drumming). But caloric burn is not the only benefit we get from fidgeting, and here we come to its second purpose. There is something about prolonged sitting that is so deeply harmful for our health that it doesn't even get rehabilitated much by the activity afterwards. There is a clear association between extensive sedentary time and its negative effects on cardiovascular and metabolic health. Studies show high glucose and insulin levels in people spending long hours sitting at their desks. Remember lipoprotein lipase, an enzyme that breaks down fats in the bloodstream? After a few hours of sitting these enzymes start switching off, and by the end of the day their activity drops by 50%. Weakened muscles, stiffened joints, general fatigue – all this is not unfamiliar to folks with sitting jobs.

The good news is it doesn't take much to improve the glycemic response and negate other negative outcomes; short breaks with light to moderate activity significantly reduce cardiovascular risk and lower glucose and insulin levels. We are talking about 1-2 minutes walks that break up sitting every 30 minutes. Remarkably, even these brief interruptions with such a light activity as walking turned out to be more beneficial than longer planned ones, two 15-minute breaks per workday. This emphasizes the point that it's not just the total amount of activity that is important – it's the very fact of breaking up prolonged uninterrupted sitting that brings maximum benefit. This brings us back to this all-important role of fidgeting – it's very effective way of doing just that, eliminating long periods of immobility.

Most forms of exercise traditionally focus on endurance and strength, making cardio and resistance training major parts of planned physical activity. Often overlooked are **flexibility** and **balance**. That's unfortunate since they play a large role in maintaining our agility as we age.

It is not my intent to make this book am exercising guide, so I will limit myself to brief descriptions of the ways to proceed, in the hopes of nudging you in the right direction. Considering their popularity of late, there is a good chance that you already engage in, or at least are well aware of, two major ways to improve those sides of your physical well-being.

One of course is yoga. No matter what your current level of flexibility is, you will benefit hugely from practicing it in the form and to the extent of your ability. There is no need to tie yourself in pretzel or do a headstand; there are poses and breathing exercises suiting any age or physical fitness level. Make sure that you pick those that stretch all major parts of your body, combining them in a single workout. Do them slowly, deliberately and thoughtfully, controlling your form and breathing. If you are very pressed for time and have to pick just a few, do a hero pose, a downward-facing dog and a cobra pose – even with all their variations they won't take more than 7-8 minutes, and you'll be amazed by how much better you feel when you finish.

Another is Tai Chi, providing many powerful health benefits. Low impact slow movements combined with deep breathing promote cardiovascular fitness, improve balance and coordination, and help lower blood pressure. Consisting of sequences of movements resembling various animal actions, it's an exercise better learned visually. Consider watching videos to learn the sequences, or better yet, join a class in your area.

These ancient practices well deserve their wide popularity, challenging the total body in ways that traditional exercise doesn't provide.

Here is how I structure my entire exercise routine. I do HIIT on the stationary bike three times a week. I add resistance training five-six days a week, alternating groups of exercise targeting the lower and upper body. I schedule upper body exercises for days coinciding with HIIT, so I don't overwork my legs with both kinds of exercises on the same day. I do some yoga at various times, here and there, as I feel the need to stretch, without designating specific time slot for it. Sometimes I just throw a few yoga positions together with a resistance workout. All that is intermixed with regular walking and fidgeting. The latter is not second nature for me so I constantly remind myself to do it. If for some reason I can't do much exercising on a particular day or week, I don't sweat it too much. Most of weight loss or maintenance is achieved through eating the right way. That said, I make sure that any pause, whatever the cause may be, doesn't stretch for too long so I don't turn into a sloth.

Maintenance Mode

When you have reached your desired weight, you switch to the maintenance mode – a regime that helps you keep off what you've lost.

It's impossible to overestimate the importance of this stage. First of all, the right strategy at this point in your journey will prevent you from returning to the same harmful behaviors and actions that got you in trouble in the first place. The last thing you want is to find yourself back where you started before implementing the strategies in this book – overweight, out of shape, ailed by illnesses. I believe you are too proud of your achievement and too happy with your newfound, lean, energetic, youthful self to let all that slip away.

Secondly, this is the mode in which you will spend the rest of life. Thus, it's vital that it's a sustainable regimen that doesn't overburden you. Not only should it be easy – it should even be easier than the weight loss mode. It should be fun, not a bore. Very importantly, it should be flexible – the rest of your life is a long time, during which you will encounter different circumstances, and your routine must be highly adaptable to see you through the vagaries of life.

Luckily, our maintenance mode is all that.

Now is a good time to summarize my experience with different flavors of the Intermittent Fasting since some of them have their use in Maintenance Mode.

- 24 hours fast ending with full sized meal
  is suitable for an experienced faster; I can
  recommend it as an occasional tool after a
  period of excess (think all-you-can-eat buffet,
  all-inclusive cruise vacation, Christmas party)
  or as a permanent fixture in your eating
  regimen once or twice a week, depending on
  the feel and need. This variation is also perfect
  for the situation where you have difficulty
  finding decent food; let's say a long flight with
  a few layovers. It's very liberating to know
  that you can cut the leash of dependency on
  whatever food you can find and simply use
  such occasion as a fasting day; just make sure
  that you have plenty of water handy. I don't
  believe it's a good idea to start your fasting
  journey with this particular modification
  though – you need to train your body to deal
  with hunger first.
- 24 hour fast ending with 500/600 calories is
  equally doable for the same purpose; during
  maintenance mode I would use it once a week.
- 16/8 can be done as a permanent eating
  schedule, or thrown in the mix with any other,
  regularly or on occasion; it's one of the easiest
  ways to maintain your target weight, especially
  when coupled with exercise in the morning.
- I still dislike "every other day" arrangement
  (eat for one day, fast for another) or a very
  low calorie every day diet. I find both overly
  restrictive and a recipe for misery. Luckily,

maintenance mode doesn't call for either of these two variations. There is one exception to the "every other day" modification though: if you need to make drastic correction to your weight (say, rectify that same cruise vacation damage) and you are now managing hunger with ease (which is all but certain after a few months on 5/2), fasting every other day for a week or two can take you to your target weight in a hurry.

- Finally, my preferred regime with which feels most comfortable upon trying all of them is a combo of 16/8 and 5/2 for the weight loss mode; 5/2 changes to 6/1 for the maintenance mode.

Let me describe this regimen as it stands after reaching my desired weight. Most of the days I fast 16 hours and then eat my daily calorie allocation during the remaining 8, usually between 1 PM and 9 PM. Do notice that this is not a requirement for the maintenance mode; I do it simply because I like this eating pattern. When you come to this point, you may very well discover that you enjoy one of IF variations, as indeed many other followers of this approach did. If I don't want to wait for my break-fast until 1 PM on a particular day, or it doesn't fit in my schedule on that day, no sweat – I go with the flow and don't think twice about it. In any case, one rule I break only very rarely: I do not snack between the meals. Contrary to popular advice, snacks keeping insulin levels constantly elevated is a recipe for increased insulin resistance resulting in a long-term disastrous consequences.

I try to keep my daily intake around 2000 calories but that's a very rough target as I don't count them regularly or weigh things I eat. Nor do I monitor the composition of my food too closely; I am satisfied by a general sense of the ratio of the macronutrients which I try to keep at 1 part protein to 2 parts fat to 1 part carbs – again, very roughly. I consider eating high quality whole foods more important than counting every gram of each of the macronutrients and I don't sweat their exact ratios or precise calorie count. If that ratio doesn't look right to you, don't think too much of it – different body types, genetic makeup and fitness goals influence these things to a large degree. This is not something to stress about or start calculating each meal. Just make sure all necessary categories are included and none of them overtakes the others by too wide margin. Also, don't be afraid of cycling through various ratios depending on season, availability and whatnot. Such cyclical variations can be just as beneficial as cycling through the fed and fasted state.

Along these lines, I make sure that my diet includes good fats (fish, butter, nuts, olive and coconut oil, meat) and avoids bad ones (chips, jams, jellies, highly processed snacks, fast foods, packaged foods). Proteins include legumes high in fiber, like black beans and chickpea, in a form of pasta, flours or beans themselves. My carbs are heavy on complex ones (buckwheat, lentils, beans, peas, fibrous vegetables, whole grains, fruits and berries) and light (very light) on simple ones (white rice, white bread, refined flours). Sweets are not excluded (far be it from me to live without a good cake or pastry!) but watched closely and consumed sparingly. I pay attention to food combinations in a single meal, making sure that I don't eat carbs or sweets alone – they are always accompanied by protein, fat and/or fiber. I also time my meals so that fruits, sweets and simple carbs are consumed around physical exertion and for the most part concentrated in the first half of the day. None of that requires much attention as it mostly became just a habit.

Once a week as a rule I do a fasting day with 600 calories. I schedule it without any firm pattern – it's simply a matter of convenience and desire (yes, the desire to fast now and then is there – that's how good it feels). As discussed earlier in this part, it's mostly a protein/fiber day, with little to no carbs and no sweets. Most often I have two meals, breaking them down as 450 and 150 calories. Sometimes it's three meals as 150-300-150 calories – it's mostly a matter of the mood of the day.

Now, I said "as a rule." That means that my guide here is the bathroom scale. If my weight remains steady and I feel great, if I had no situations or events that led to overeating, I might skip a week and enjoy my normal eating. If I had such an event or if I see my weight starting to uptick, I can throw in second fasting day a week. Alternatively, now and then I can apply one of the variations of the Intermittent Fasting we discussed earlier. It's a natural and easy balancing act where you just keep an eye on your weight and regulate it lightly. There is no heavy hand involved, no strict limitations and, within a reason, no forbidden foods.

Whatever schedule change or event life throws at you, the flexibility of this approach is truly unparalleled. Nothing prevents you from adding a fasting day, canceling it, planning it in advance or moving it to another date at a moment's notice. It can even be canceled during the fasting day, right then and there if something unexpected happens, and there won't be any harm done – you simply do it tomorrow. Let's say, you started your fast and the phone rang. It's a classmate you haven't seen in 25 years, who just landed at your city airport, and is eager to see you and reminisce about old times – naturally, over a few drinks and bar snacks. Do you sigh and say "Oh, I would love to but I fast today?" Well, you could use it as an excuse if he was the one who ratted you out to the principal for smoking in Grade 9, but providing you are glad to see him, cancel your fast and don't give it a second thought – there is always tomorrow.

There is also nothing stopping you from doing some preventive repair in case of foreseen damage. Christmas season, with a few parties and gatherings, can be preceded by a few fasting days as well as followed by them. The same can be done with that cruise with an overabundance of food freely available at every turn.

So there you go: your newly minted lifestyle laid out for you. No, it doesn't include lying on the sofa for days eating chocolate cake topped with whipped cream and washed down with a 2-litre bottle of soda. Sorry. That was the deal from the get-go – no return to the old harmful ways, but a return to an enjoyable and sustainable lifestyle instead. What it does entail is regular weigh-ins, monitoring your weight and taking measures if it shows signs of nudging upward. Those measures are well-familiar, present no great burden and most likely constitute a pleasant part of your routine by now.

What do you get in return? A lot. Great shape, good moods, marvelous food, potentially decreased or no medications, a longer and healthier life. Considering that what you have to do for all that is not in the least disagreeable, it's a wonder that this whole arrangement is even legal. I certainly find it highly acceptable. I view it as a second shot at a healthy life; having squandered my first chance and needing to work hard to undo the damage, there is no way I am going to waste my second, and probably last shot.

This book is your personal invitation and a map to this thrilling and highly rewarding journey. It is my sincere hope that you accept this invitation and use this map to chart your course.

There is a lot more to discuss and share on this exciting path. Please come to http://timetraveldiet.com/ for more topics and recipes, to follow my next steps and share your stories and discoveries. Let's continue this journey together. Let's reshape the way we eat. I am interested to hear your insights, answer your questions, take part in troubleshooting your steps and applaud your success stories.

Resources

Starting Point

Most common unit conversions in this book:

1 kg = 2.2 pounds

1 pound = 0,454 kg

1 litre = 1.06 quart = 2.1 pint = 34 ounce

Fahrenheit to Celsius conversion for recipes: http://www.metric-conversions.org/temperature/fahrenheit-to-celsius.htm

Conversion of Glucose Values from mg/dl to mmol/l: http://www.soc-bdr.org/rds/authors/unit_tables_conversions_and_genetic_dictionaries/e5184/index_en.html

Discussion of a possibility of the Type 2 Diabetes reversal:
http://www.webmd.com/diabetes/type-2-diabetes-guide/reversing-type-2-diabetes

Defining "remission" or "cure" by American Diabetes Association:
http://care.diabetesjournals.org/content/32/11/2133
https://www.ncbi.nlm.nih.gov/pmc/articles/PMC2768219/

New perspectives on the diabetes reversal by Roy Taylor, MD:
http://care.diabetesjournals.org/content/36/4/1047?i-jkey=742f55dac3653a6ceab5cef28bcf86d9bb93f-d35&keytype2=tf_ipsecsha

Smart BMI calculator going a bit beyond many standard ones. It takes age and sex into account and estimates the significance of your indication for your health:
http://www.smartbmicalculator.com/

Minus Sugar
Close look at the popular drinks caloric count and sugar content:
http://globalnews.ca/news/2739686/
how-much-sugar-and-how-many-calories-are-in-your-summertime-drink/

Studies showing positive correlation between artificial sweetener use and weight gain:
https://www.ncbi.nlm.nih.gov/pmc/articles/
PMC2892765/

"Routine consumption of diet soft drinks is linked to increases in the same risks that many seek to avoid by using artificial sweeteners—namely type 2 diabetes, metabolic syndrome heart disease, and stroke:"
https://www.ncbi.nlm.nih.gov/pmc/articles/
PMC4883499/

Coffee and caffeinated tea associated with a lower T2D (when consumed unsweetened):
https://www.ncbi.nlm.nih.gov/pubmed/23151535/

What is parboiled rice:
https://en.wikipedia.org/wiki/Parboiled_rice

Benefits of parboiled rice:
http://healthyeating.sfgate.com/benefits-par-boiled-rice-7618.html

Basics and health benefits of buckwheat:
http://wholegrainscouncil.org/whole-grains-101/easy-ways-enjoy-whole-grains/grain-month-calendar/buckwheat-december-grain-month

Resistant starches: what they are, how they help, where they reside etc:
https://chriskresser.com/how-resistant-starch-will-help-to-make-you-healthier-and-thinner/
http://www.marksdailyapple.com/the-definitive-guide-to-resistant-starch/
http://www.marksdailyapple.com/resistant-starch-your-questions-answered/

Resistant starch positive influence on metabolic responses:
https://www.ncbi.nlm.nih.gov/pubmed/15287677

Health properties of resistant starch, content in various foods, physiological effects, effects on short-chain fatty acids and colonic function, lipid profile etc.; review of the studies:
http://onlinelibrary.wiley.com/
doi/10.1111/j.1467-3010.2005.00481.x/full

Large database of resistant starch content in various foods:
http://freetheanimal.com/wp-content/uploads/2013/08/
Resistant-Starch-in-Foods.pdf

Recipes with konnyaku (shirataki):
http://recipesfortom.blogspot.ca/2011/09/konnyaku.
html

Second meal effect: how it helps reduce glycemic responses:
http://www.omicsonline.org/the-second-meal-effect-
and-its-influence-on-glycemia-2161-0509.1000108.
php?aid=4874
http://images.abbottnutrition.com/ANHI/MEDIA/
Second%20Meal%20Effect%20Review%20and%20
Citation%20Table.pdf

Guidelines to using flours other than wheat:
http://www.forkandbeans.com/2013/12/30/
guide-gluten-free-flours/
http://potluck.ohmyveggies.com/
beginners-guide-gluten-free-flours/

Plus Bacteria

Benefits of fermented foods for health:
http://onlinelibrary.wiley.com/
doi/10.1111/j.1365-2672.2006.02963.x/full

How to Fix Your Gut Bacteria and Lose Weight:
http://drhyman.com/blog/2016/02/18/
how-to-fix-your-gut-bacteria-and-lose-weight/

Website and book by world renowned fermentation
expert Sandor Katz:
http://www.wildfermentation.com/
http://www.wildfermentation.com/wild-fermentation/

There is no other book incorporating sauerkraut in
all kinds of meals like this one: Fresh & Fermented: 85
Delicious Ways to Make Fermented Carrots, Kraut, and
Kimchi Part of Every Meal by Julie O'Brien:
https://www.amazon.ca/Fresh-
Fermented-Delicious-Carrots-Kimchi/
dp/1570619379
https://www.amazon.com/Fresh-Fermented-
Delicious-Carrots-Kimchi-ebook/dp/
B00K4BA8HU

It's not a coincidence that I suggest cinnamon in many
recipes, nor is it purely for its taste. It has positive influence on fasting blood sugar and lipids:
https://www.ncbi.nlm.nih.gov/
pubmed/?term=Davis+Yokoyama+Cinnamon
https://www.ncbi.nlm.nih.gov/pubmed/22749176
https://www.ncbi.nlm.nih.gov/pubmed/17556692

In case you can't source kombucha SCOBY, how to grow your own:
https://www.youtube.com/watch?v=F3TN54s_ezA

Positive effect of kefir on glycemic control:
https://www.ncbi.nlm.nih.gov/pubmed/25905057
https://www.ncbi.nlm.nih.gov/pubmed/26732026

If you are worried about using full fat diary, don't. Review of 29 studies shows absence of weight loss effect caused by it:
https://www.ncbi.nlm.nih.gov/pubmed/22932282

... And another study shows full-fat diary decreases insulin levels and risk of diabetes:
https://www.ncbi.nlm.nih.gov/pmc/articles/PMC3056495/

... and if that's not enough, Foods rich in protein, dairy products help dieters preserve muscle and lose belly fat:
http://jn.nutrition.org/content/141/9/1626.full%22%3EJournal%20of%20Nutrition

Comparison of kefir and yogurt health benefits:
http://www.culturesforhealth.com/learn/milk-kefir/difference-between-kefir-yogurt/
http://www.theglobeandmail.com/life/health-and-fitness/ask-a-health-expert/whats-the-difference-between-yogurt-and-kefir/article7904569/

Microbiological and therapeutic properties of kefir:
https://www.ncbi.nlm.nih.gov/pmc/articles/
PMC3833126/

Multiple ways to use whey:
http://dontwastethecrumbs.com/2014/05/36-ways-to-
use-whey-and-5-ways-to-make-it/
http://www.farmcurious.com/blogs/
farmcurious/17599408-cheesemaking-what-to-do-with-
all-that-whey

Making ricotta cheese from whey:
http://www.culturesforhealth.com/learn/recipe/
cheese-recipes/whey-traditional-ricotta-cheese/

One more link for the fermented buckwheat bread with
additional details:
http://phickle.com/
gluten-free-sourdough-buckwheat-bread-recipe/

As we discuss healthy desserts, ice cream in particular,
I'd like to show you what you are actually getting with
many popular ice cream choices from the store shelf:
http://globalnews.ca/news/2793880/
how-much-sugar-and-how-many-calories-are-in-your-
summertime-ice-cream/

Minus Pounds
Metabolic changes at different times during fasting:
http://io9.gizmodo.com/5941883/how-your-body-fights-
to-keep-you-alive-when-youre-starving

Overview of fasting with diabetes, comparison of blood glucose and insulin levels under low fat, low carb and IF diets:
https://www.fastday.com/fasting/
fasting-with-medical-conditions/fasting-with-diabetes/

A few popular beliefs about obesity and weight loss strategies that are actually nothing more than myths:
http://www.nejm.org/doi/full/10.1056/
NEJMsa1208051#t=articleBackground

Intermittent fasting basics, includes plenty of links to studies:
https://authoritynutrition.com/
intermittent-fasting-guide/

Fasting for weight loss:
http://globalnews.ca/news/2572885/fasting-for-weight-loss-heres-why-scientists-says-it-works-long-term/

FAQ about fasting answered by Michael Mosley. Entire website is highly informative, and the book The Fast Diet is a valuable resource.
https://thefastdiet.co.uk/
michael-answers-frequently-asked-questions/

Exercise effect on Type 2 Diabetics:
https://www.ncbi.nlm.nih.gov/pubmed/16855995

Effect of walking on glycemic control and weight loss in diabetics:
https://diatribe.org/issues/51/adams-corner
https://www.ncbi.nlm.nih.gov/pubmed/17224062/
https://www.ncbi.nlm.nih.gov/pmc/articles/
PMC3302145/

... and healthy persons:
https://www.ncbi.nlm.nih.gov/pubmed/12665983
http://www.nature.com/ijo/journal/v24/n10/
full/0801399a.html

Dangers of prolonged sitting (hint: there are many, including but not limited to increased blood pressure, high blood sugar, excess body fat around the waist and abnormal cholesterol levels):
http://www.mayoclinic.org/healthy-lifestyle/
adult-health/expert-answers/sitting/faq-20058005
http://www.aafp.org/news/health-of-the-pub-
lic/20150127sitting.html

How breaking up prolonged sitting improves blood sugar and insulin response:
https://www.ncbi.nlm.nih.gov/pmc/articles/
PMC3329818/
https://www.ncbi.nlm.nih.gov/pubmed/26628415
https://www.ncbi.nlm.nih.gov/pmc/articles/
PMC4995540/

Fidgeting effect on weight loss:
https://www.theguardian.com/lifeandstyle/1999/
feb/23/healthandwellbeing.health
https://www.ncbi.nlm.nih.gov/pubmed/15681386
https://www.ncbi.nlm.nih.gov/pubmed/9880251
Positive effects of High Intensity Interval Training on
blood sugar and insulin resistance:
http://onlinelibrary.wiley.com/doi/10.1111/obr.12317/
abstract

... And on blood pressure:
http://www.mayoclinicproceedings.org/article/
S0025-6196(11)61303-7/abstract

Why traditional cardio exercise is not an effective
weight loss strategy:
http://www.leanerbydesign.com/
cardio-poor-value-money-comes-fat-loss/

Basics of Tabata Protocol:
http://www.tabataprotocol.com/

You Are Your Own Gym: The Bible of Bodyweight
Exercises Paperback by Mark Lauren
https://www.amazon.com/gp/product/0345528581/
https://www.amazon.ca/You-Are-Your-Own-Gym/
dp/0345528581

Many ways to do a plank:
http://www.health.com/health/gallery/0,,20813896,00.
html/view-all

Health effects of Tai Chi:
http://www.health.harvard.edu/staying-healthy/
the-health-benefits-of-tai-chi

The Obesity Code: Unlocking the Secrets of Weight Loss
by Dr. Jason Fung:
https://www.amazon.ca/
Obesity-Code-Unlocking-Secrets-Weight/dp/1771641258
https://www.amazon.com/
Obesity-Code-Unlocking-Secrets-Weight/dp/1771641258

Interview with Dr. Fung:
http://www.drfranklipman.
com/q-dr-jason-fung-book-obesity-code/
https://www.thestar.com/life/
health_wellness/2016/01/25/scarborough-doctors-book-
says-insulin-makes-you-fat-fasting-makes-you-thin.
html

Acknowledgments

This book is largely a friends-and-family affair. As such, major thanks go to those who suffered the most through both the weight loss journey and writing the book about it.

My wife Iryna, for courageously making herself a willing subject of all the experiments.

My daughter Olga, Nutrition and Dietetics MScA candidate at McGill University, for help with research and for critical feedback on my ideas.

My son Ilya and his wife Katrina, for patiently listening to my ruminations about the endless twists and turns in the story, and for all the work with editing my writing.

My grandson Niko for providing endless inspiration to stay healthy and watch him grow.

My long-time friend through thick and thin, Mark Ierardo, for enormous help with editing the book and, of course, for keeping my feet planted on the ground with his skeptical pragmatism.

The best book designer in town and friend, Iryna Spica, for all the work on the book cover and layout, and hours-long discussions of all the aspects of publishing.

To all my friends who followed my trials and errors, providing encouragement, fearlessly tasting my culinary creations and serving as sounding boards for my musings about my experiences and the next steps.

Index